BEAUTY AND COSMETICS IN THE TIME OF JANE AUSTEN

SARAH JANE DOWNING

AMBERLEY

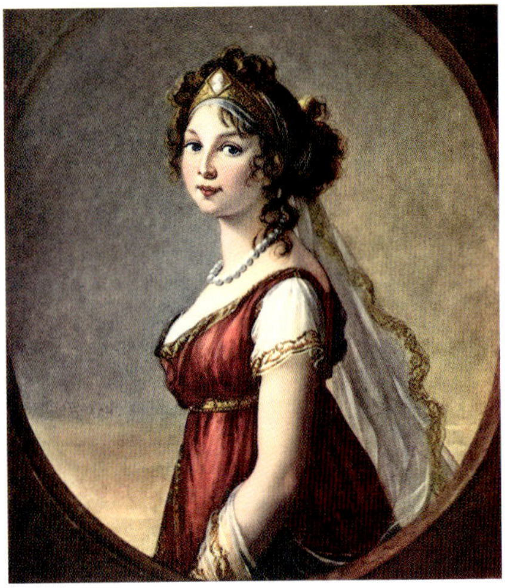

Front cover: 'L'Enfant au Fard' (Louis Léopold Boilly, *c*. 1795); *back cover*: 'Le Lever des Grizettes' (Le Bon Genre, *c*. 1800).

Left: Queen Louise Augusta of Prussia (Elisabeth Vigée Le Brun, 1802). Neoclassical hairstyle of ringlets and Greco-Roman-style tiara.

First published 2025

Amberley Publishing
The Hill, Stroud,
Gloucestershire, GL5 4EP

www.amberley-books.com

ISBN: 978 1 3981 2313 7 (print)
ISBN: 978 1 3981 2314 4 (ebook)

British Library Cataloguing in Publication Data.
A catalogue record for this book is available from the British Library.

Typeset in 10pt on 13pt Celeste.
Typesetting by SJmagic DESIGN SERVICES, India.
Printed in the UK.

Appointed GPSR EU Representative: Easy Access System Europe Oü, 16879218
Address: Mustamäe tee 50, 10621, Tallinn, Estonia
Contact Details: gpsr.requests@easproject.com, +358 40 500 3575

Contents

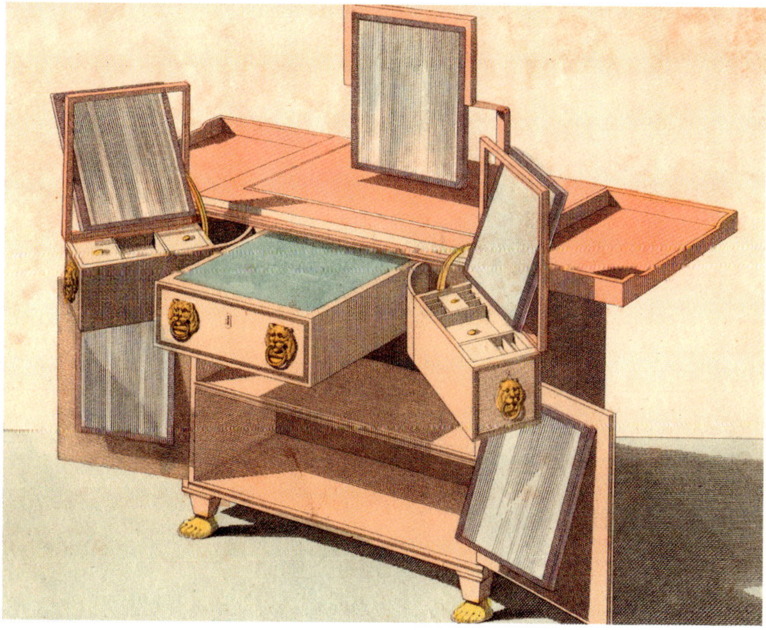

'The Ladies Toilet Dressing Case' (Ackermann's *Repository of Arts,* 1812). As well as multiple angled mirrors that fold away there is a writing drawer that pulls out.

Introduction

When Jane Austen was born on 16 December 1775 the world was on the brink of revolution. The battle for American independence heralded an era of revolutionary ideas that would see the old order swept away across Europe in a tide of revolution and war. Although few women were directly involved in determining the new paths taken by politics, war and industry, their lives, their beauty and their fashions were nevertheless irreversibly changed.

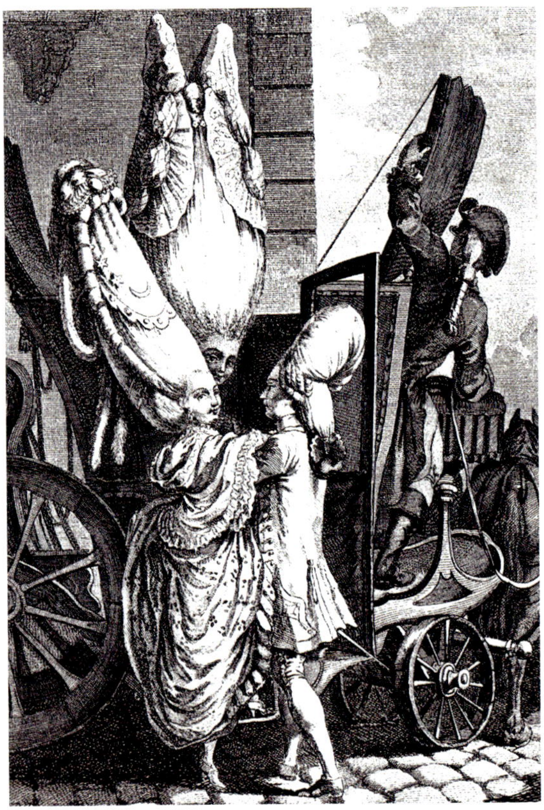

Getting into the coach, *c.* 1770. Hair was so high during the 1770s that carriages had to be adapted to accommodate it.

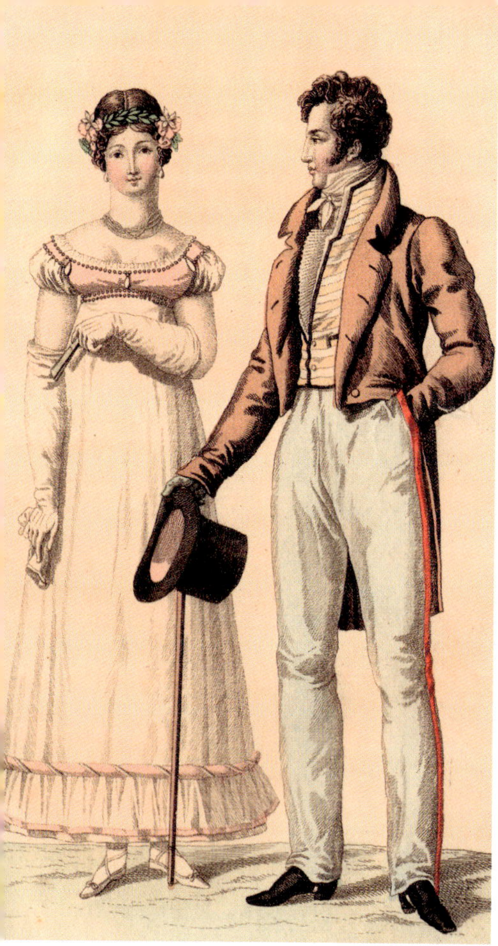

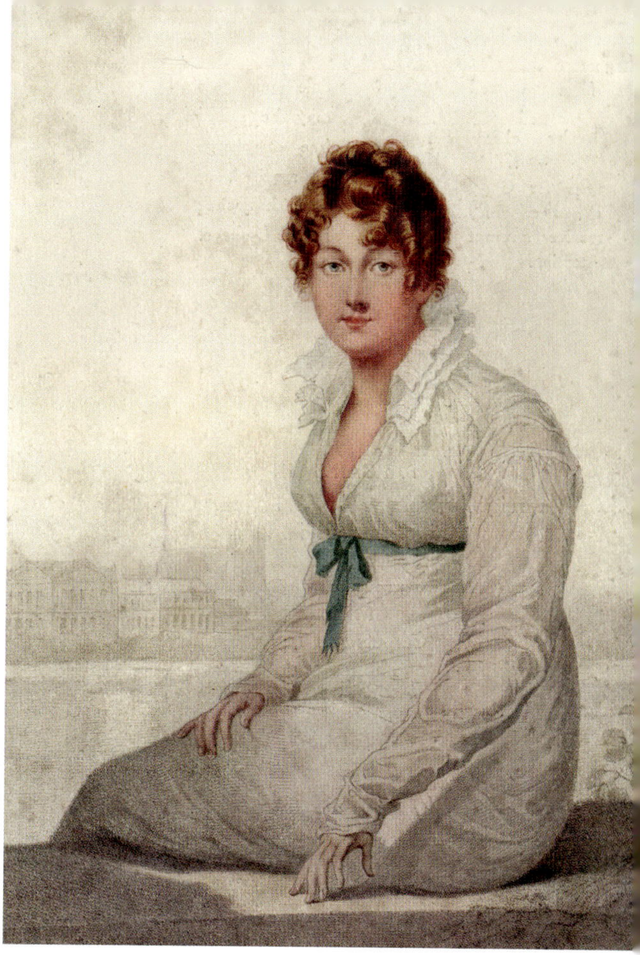

Above left: 'Costumes Parisiens', 1815. The epitome of the modern couple.

Above right: *Portrait of Mrs. Q* (Mrs Harriet Quentin) by François Huet-Villiers. Jane saw this portrait at an exhibition in Spring Gardens and in her letter of 24 May 1813 she wrote of her character in *Pride and Prejudice*: 'Mrs Bingley is exactly herself, size, shaped face, features & sweetness; there never was a greater likeness.'

Towering Frenched hairstyles and lead-based cosmetics were exchanged for pearl powder, vegetable rouge and glossy ringlets, and fashion documented the changes as silks, velvets and brocades were exchanged for muslin, cotton and broadcloth. These democratic choices represented a renunciation of the old order, where the French court had dictated fashion for all. Gone were the highly decorative rigid costumes of courtly display, banished in favour of the insouciant riding breeches, boots and redingote of Beau Brummel and the high-waisted free skirt and flat shoe of Elizabeth Bennet.

Although Jane Austen rarely mentions cosmetics, she weaves the themes of beauty, vivacity, health and 'the bloom of youth' throughout her plots, most notably in the restoration of Anne Elliot's beauty in *Persuasion*. However, Jane is always very clear that beauty comes from within, and it is Anne's restoration to herself that restores her bloom, just as it is Lizzie's clarity and self-possession that gives her hers.

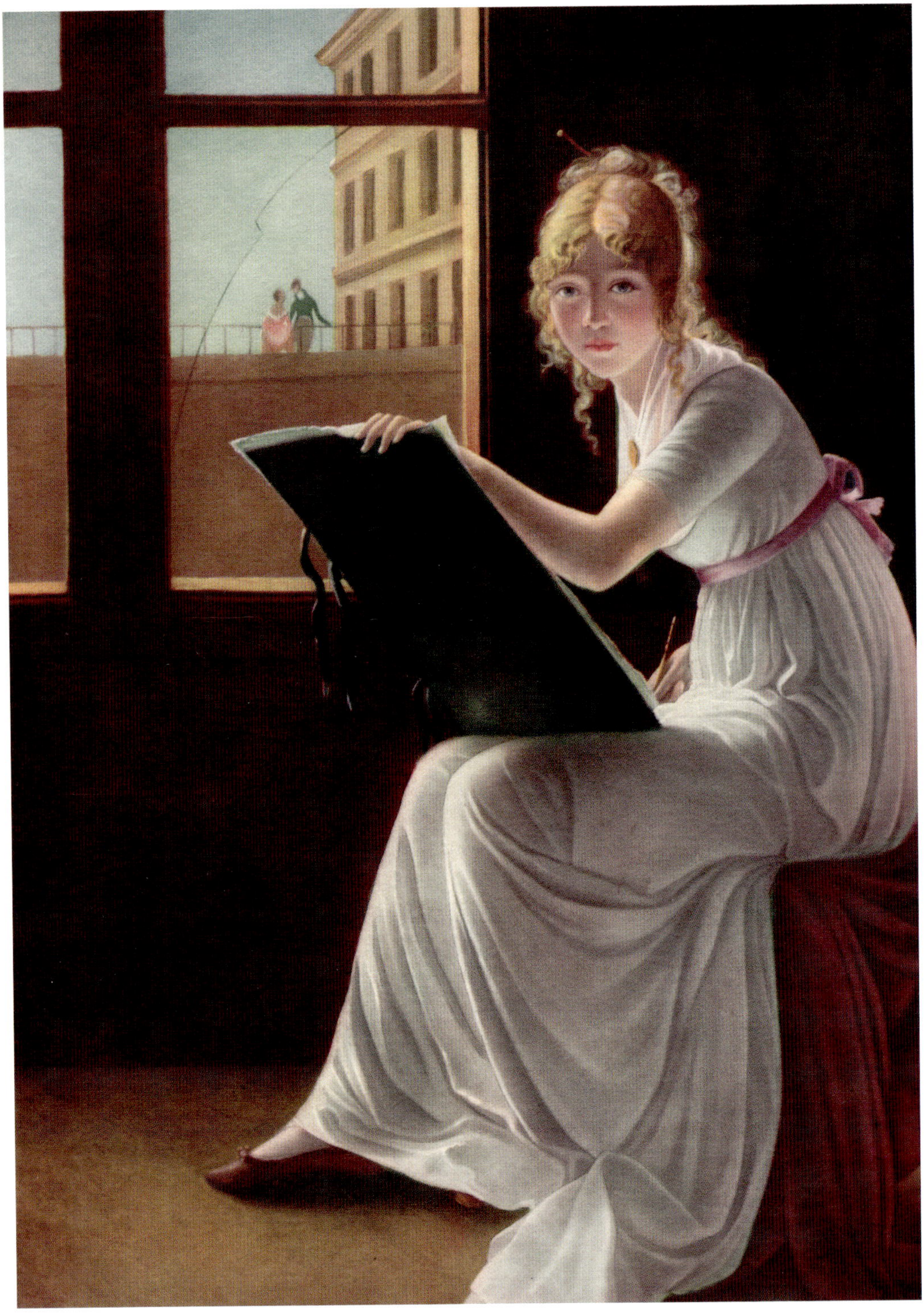

Mlle Charlotte du Val d'Ognes or *Young Woman Drawing* (Marie Denice Villers, 1801). Like Emma, 'She is loveliness itself'.

Emma Woodhouse is her most beautiful heroine: 'Can you imagine anything nearer perfect beauty than Emma altogether – face and figure? ... Such an eye! the true hazel eye – and so brilliant! regular features, open countenance, with a complexion – oh, what a bloom ... She is loveliness itself.'

It has been suggested that, as a lady who never married, Jane was frumpy, less than pretty and a rather clichéd spinster. This misconception would seem to reflect that attitudes about women and their beauty – especially older or unmarried women – have progressed very little over the last two centuries! James Edward Austen-Leigh wrote in his memoir of Jane published in 1871:

> In person she was very attractive; her figure was rather tall and slender, her step light and firm, and her whole appearance expressive of health and animation. In complexion she was a clear brunette with a rich colour; she had full round cheeks, with mouth and nose small and well formed, bright hazel eyes, and brown hair forming natural curls close round her face. If not so regularly handsome as her sister, yet her countenance had a peculiar charm of its own to the eyes of most beholders.

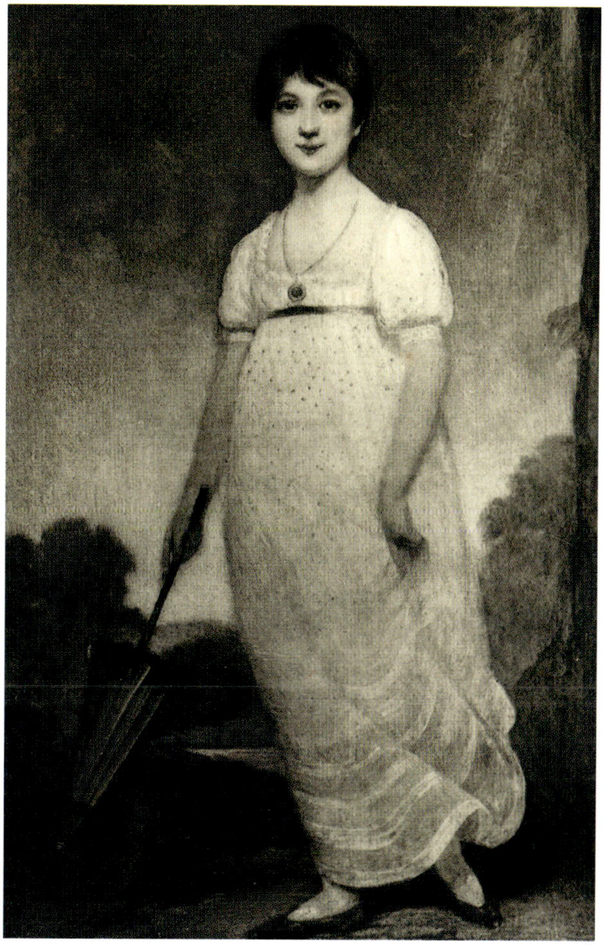

The Rice Portrait (Ozias Humphrey *c.* 1792–93). Thought to be of the young Jane Austen, aged around seventeen, it was originally held within the Austen-Knight family collection.

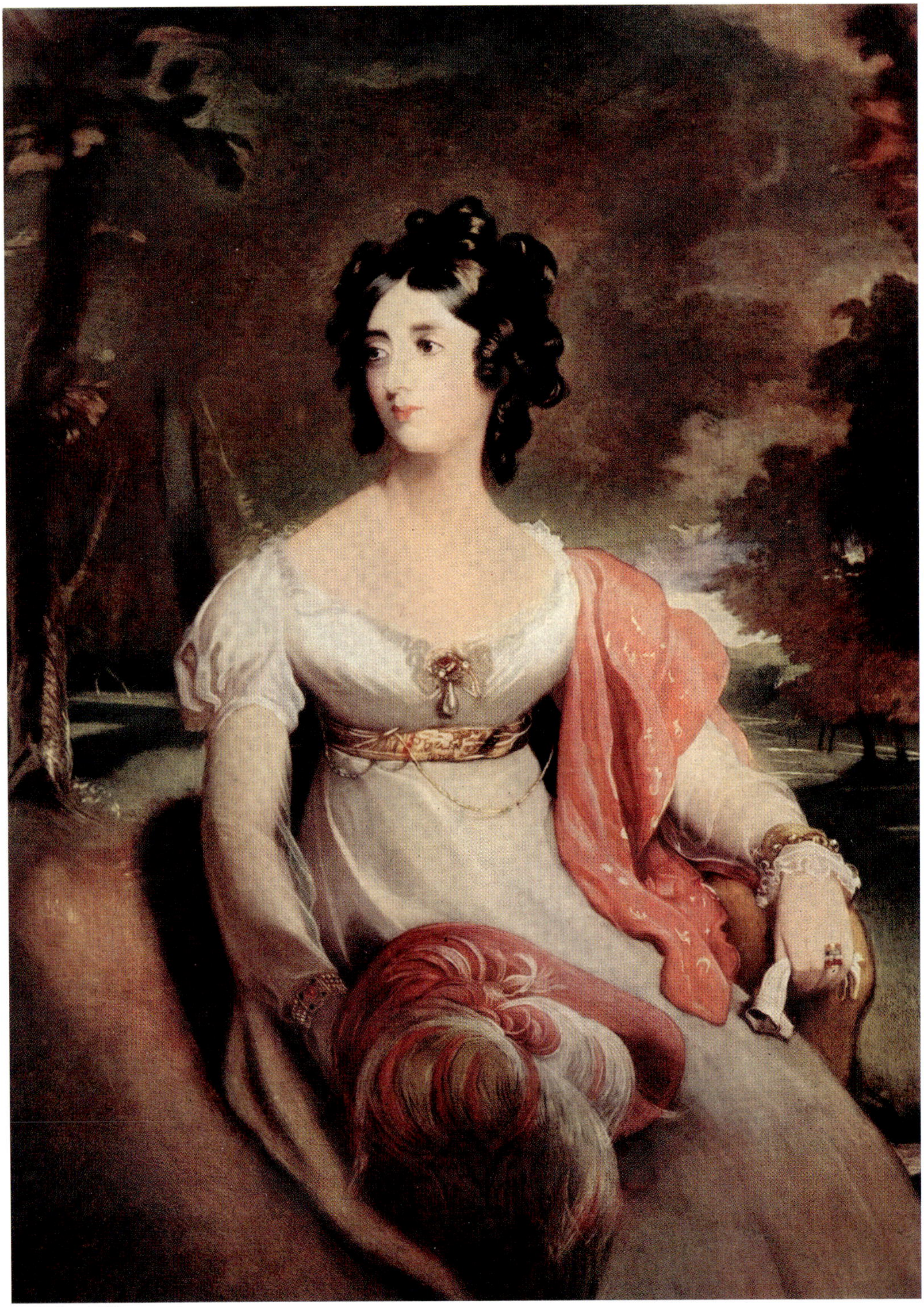

Julia, Lady Peel (Sir Thomas Lawrence, *c.* 1820). With her glossy ringlets, she was the embodiment of Regency beauty.

When Jane was making her debut at the Basingstoke assemblies in 1792, young women had to find balance on the double-edged sword of beauty; they were expected to be as natural and wholesome as possible, yet captivatingly beautiful. She was well aware that beauty was currency and that, with less currency, 'plain' girls were at a distinct disadvantage. She was also aware of the crushing notion that once a pretty girl has become a wife and mother, her life would be subsumed into those of her children and husband. A pretty young woman was an ornament to her family, a reflection of their importance that could be used to make a great alliance. She is then an ornament to her husband, helping to draw him to favourable attention, ensuring his status in the most prestigious circles. She then does the same for her children, maintaining her beauty more subtly, but enough to reassure any potential suitors to her daughters that they will still be attractive and appropriate even into advanced maturity – beyond the age of thirty!

For many women their beauty was no more their own than their lives were. Little could be done about the obligations and strictures upon a female life, but a woman could develop her own beauty for herself. Her beauty could be found in her warm, loving smile, in the light of playful wit dancing in her eyes and her graceful step as she dances. It could be found in her passion for literature and poetry, in her bright and lively mind, or in her joy as she strides out through the countryside – mud be damned! In her novels, Jane has developed a depth of beauty for her characters that goes way beyond a pretty figure and a fresh complexion, a true spirit of beauty that reaches across the centuries to touch us heart and soul.

I

What Went Before and Other Excesses

Jane was only eleven when she first met her 'outlandish' cousin, Eliza de Feuillide, at Christmas 1786, and the glamorous countess made quite an impression on her. It has been suggested that she modelled the engaging Lady Susan from the titular novel after her, as well as the lovely Mary Crawford in *Mansfield Park* as they each shared a love of amateur theatricals and a prodigious talent for the harp. To be able to play the angelic instrument was the height of fashion at the French court, so as well as a wonderful opportunity to

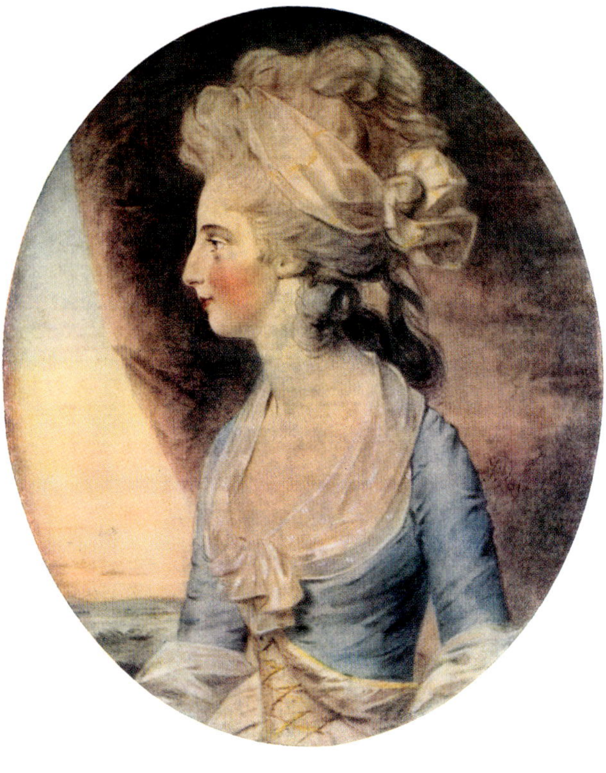

Mary Isabella, Duchess of Rutland (John Downman, *c.* 1790). The style of the duchess' hair and gown are very similar to those worn in the portrait miniature of Eliza de Feuillide. Her rouge is in the French style, reaching from eyelash to jaw line.

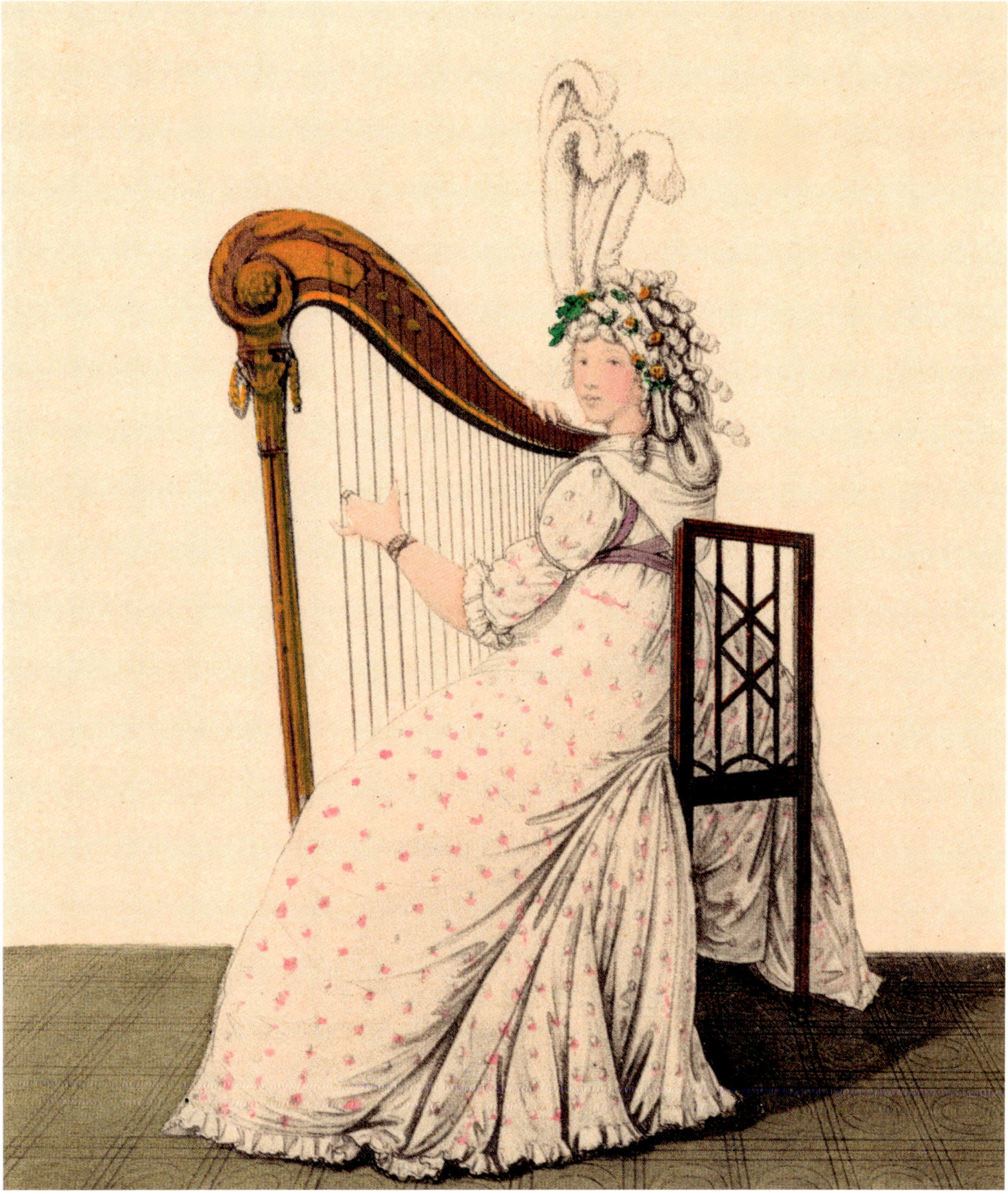

Heideloff's 'Gallery of Fashion', April 1795. She wears one of the fashionable styles of ringlets dressed with court plumes with a low chignon looped up at the back.

display elegant arms and graceful hands, mastering the instrument also made it clear that the player was well acquainted with aristocratic society.

Jane may have spent most of her time in provincial circles with few glimpses of true glamour, but as a child she had had ample time to gaze upon her pretty cousin's elfin features in the portrait miniature that she had sent to 'my Uncle G Austen' in 1780. Eliza was

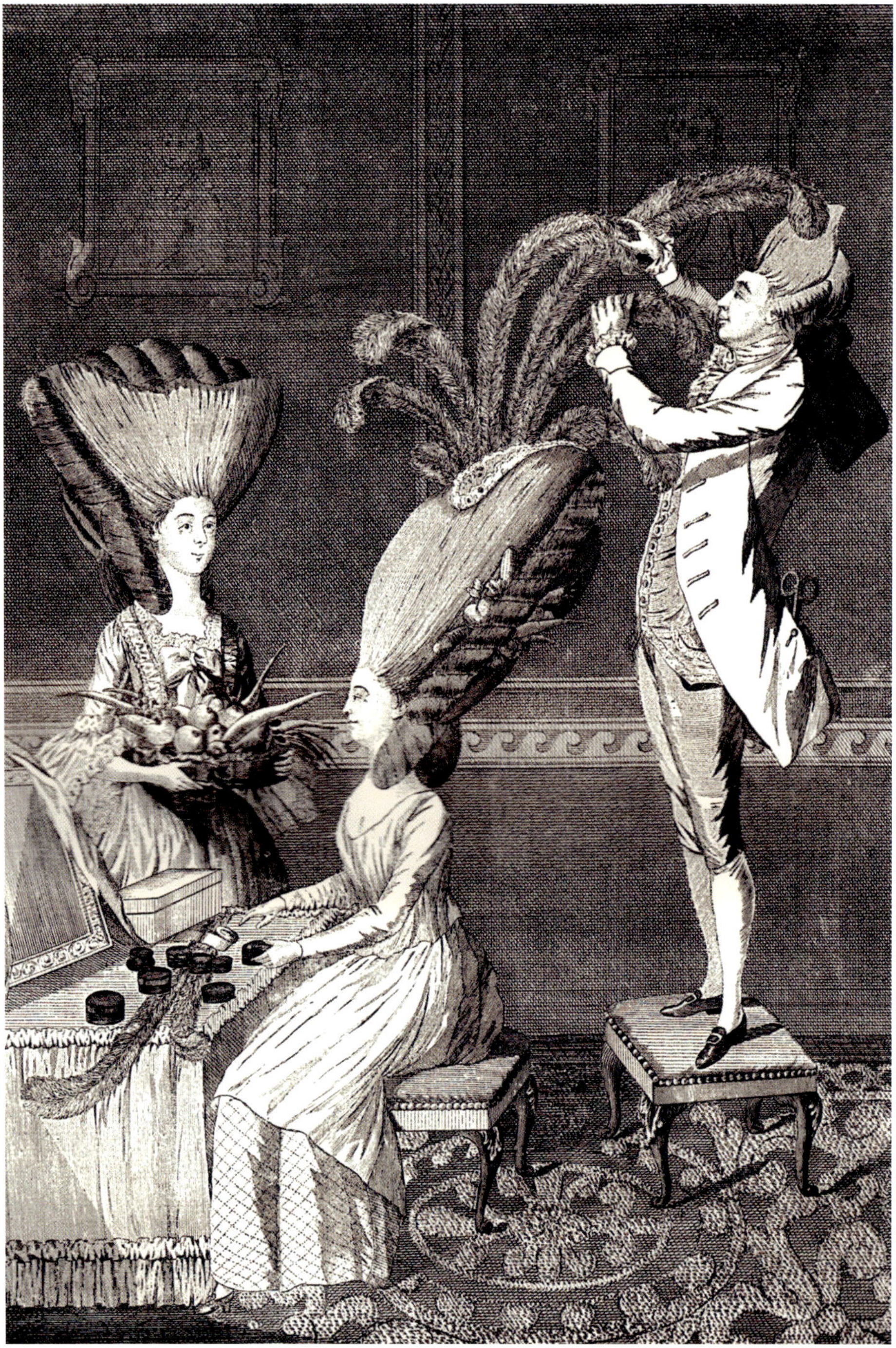

The Preposterous Head Dress or *The Feathered Lady* by Matthias Darley, 26 March 1776. Ladies and their hairdressers were very creative, using an abundance of props to curate whole scenes and themed hairstyles to commemorate events. The most famous was Marie Antoinette's *Coiffure à la Belle-Poule* which featured a ship in full rigging in celebration of the naval victory in the American War of Independence.

depicted with her hair lightly powdered in delicately dishevelled curls beribboned in blue to match those on her gown. Once engaged to the Count de Feuillide in 1781, Jane's cousin Eliza was elevated to the royal circle of the French court, and she couldn't wait to share all the details in her letters. She might well have been inspired in her beauty choices, as she noted: 'Powder is universally worn, & in very large quantities, no one would dare to appear in public without it,' adding that the queen 'had white lilac together with gauze, Feathers, ribbon and diamonds intermixed with her hair', a style not unlike that which she chose for her miniature.

Marie Antoinette and her ladies were legendary for their beauty, which Eliza was keen to confirm when she wrote to her cousin, Phylly, on 16 May 1780: 'The Queen is a very fine Woman, She has a most beautiful complexion, & is indeed exceedingly handsome ... She was without gloves, I suppose to shew her hands, & arms, which are without exception the whitest & most beautiful I ever beheld.'

Undoubtedly impressed, cousin Phylly must have enquired about cosmetics as Eliza wrote again on 27 June 1780: 'You wrong her Majesty however when you suppose her entirely indebted to art for her complexion. She has a really beautiful natural one, rouge I acknowledge is much worn here, but not so universally as you imagine.'

The pernicious effects of ceruse made of white lead had long been suspected, but its pure white was so good at concealing flaws and perfecting the slight translucent gloss of

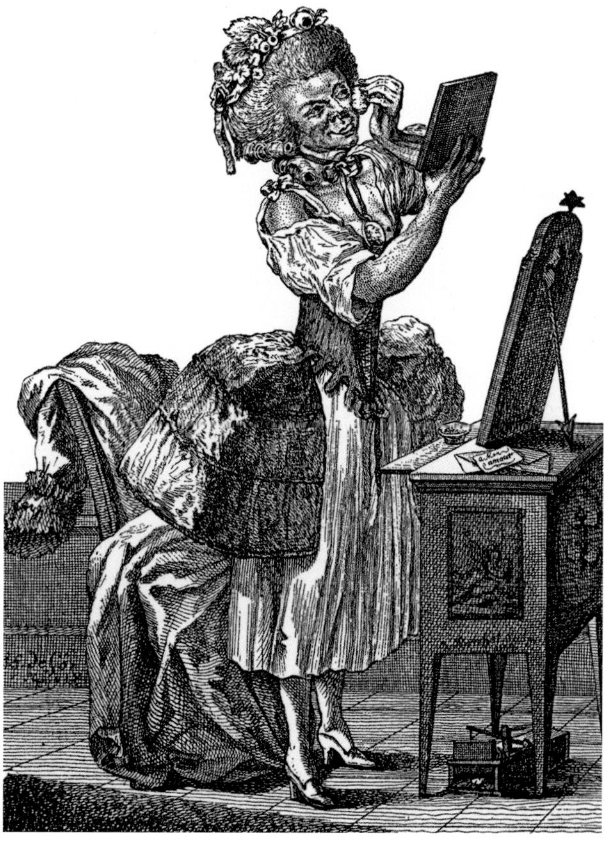

'Supplementing Faded Charms' (Joseph Franz von Goz, 1783). She has a mousetrap set under her dressing table to ensure her 'eyebrows for tomorrow'!

porcelain that looked so well against the powdered coiffure that few fashionable beauties could resist! It gave the best coverage for blemishes and the ravages of smallpox, bouts of which still frequently broke out. It created a fine base for the deep shades of mercuric rouge that had been so popular, and it would see off any unwanted facial hair. This might have been regarded as a benefit by those worried by a low forehead or a worryingly hirsute lip, but it was frequently a disaster for the eyebrows. However, as early as 1703 an ingenious solution was found – mice! These unwanted guests were in many houses and their short, silky, brown fur somehow suggested itself as the perfect material for the artificial eyebrow. The mouse hide was cut to the desired shape and glued in place, often a little higher than the natural eyebrow.

The poet Jonathan Swift wrote 'A Beautiful Young Nymph Going to Bed: Written for the Honour of the Fair Sex' (1731), including mouse-skin eyebrows as part of her catalogue of artificial aids to beauty:

Her eye-brows, from a mouse's hide,
Stuck on with art on either side,
Pulls off with care, and first displays 'em,
Then in a play-book smoothly lays 'em.

Critics of cosmetics made much of the unpleasant aspects of ceruse. According *to The Art of Beauty* (1825), one calamitous disadvantage was that the foul, sulphurous, garlic breath of a puffing dance partner or an admirer looming too close could discolour ceruse to a foreboding dark grey.

Such penalties might have been acceptable as the price of beauty, but once there began to be fatalities associated with ceruse it was difficult to continue to justify its use. In 1766, Horace Walpole reported: 'That pretty young woman, Lady Fortrose, Lady Harrington's eldest daughter, is at the point of death, killed like Lady Coventry and others, by white lead, of which nothing could break her.'

Fortunately, there were no fatalities from the extreme hairstyles that had been worn in the 1760s and 1770s, although there were a number of near misses caused when ladies lingered too long beneath low chandeliers, giving their hair – decorated with ostrich plumes sometimes over 4 feet high – time to catch light. The fashion for high Frenched hairstyles had even caused changes in carriage design as seats had to be lowered to accommodate them. All of the doorways at Versailles were also raised to the ceiling to allow women to make an entrance without stooping, and chandeliers were raised everywhere to try to avoid headdress fires. Unfortunately, at the Assembly Rooms in Bath they were loath to compromise the ambience, and a fashionable lady caught fire. Thankfully, she was extinguished in time, but her misfortune was memorialised in Christopher Anstey's 1776 satirical poem 'An Election Ball':

Yet Miss at the rooms
Must beware of her plumes;
For if Vulcan her feather embraces, Like poor Lady Laycock
She'll burn like a haycock,
And roast all the Loves and the Graces.

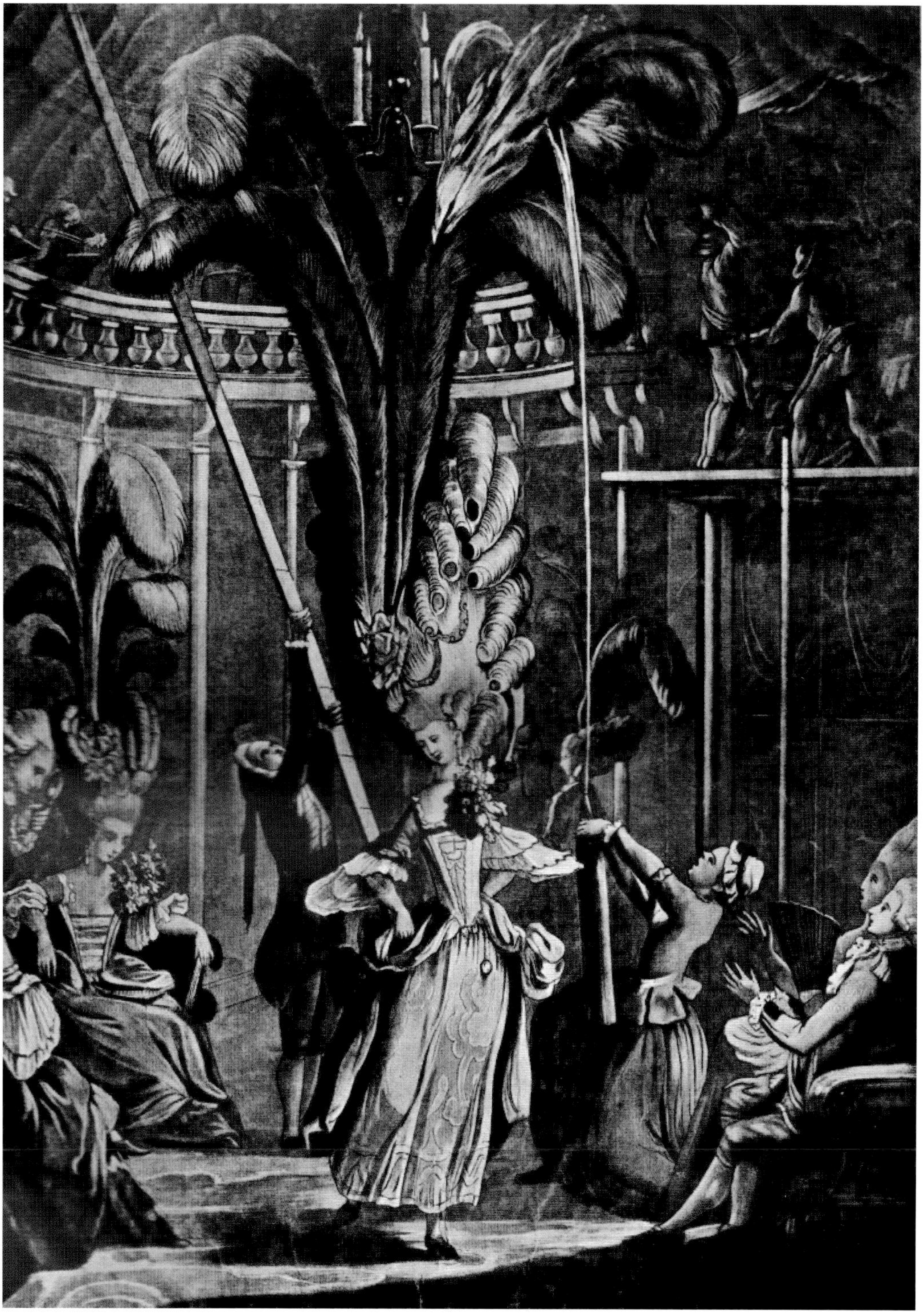

'Hints to the Ladies to Take Care of their Heads' (Sayer and Bennet, 1776). A satirical illustration of a headdress fire.

There had been a steady growth in height and intricacy of hairstyles, or *têtes*, since 1763 when Legros de Rumigny (the chef turned coiffeuse) took Paris by storm with his book *L'Encyclopedie Carcassiere, ou tableaux des coiffures a la mode gravees sur les desseins des petites-maitresses de Paris* and practically invented the concept of the professional hairdresser. He opened his Academie des Coiffures to teach the art of creating the styles. 'Hair dressers' could pay to attend professionally, but there were also less-expensive courses for maids and valets, so even provincial ladies could have their maids trained in Paris to ensure the fashionable future of their coiffures. The result was a growing professional class of hairdressers, who maintained high standards of artistry for their clients on both sides of the Channel.

However, Marie Antoinette's personal preference was for more natural styles and once she became a mother, she spent more time at Le Petit Triannon with her children, where she could follow Rousseau's newly sanctioned natural philosophies and play at being a shepherdess in the perfect pastoral idyll. Leonard designed the simpler *Coiffure a l'Enfant* for her in 1781; her hair was cut to allow the top and sides to be frizzled or creped in tight curls, with the only length to be left at the back to wear long ringlets around her shoulders. Although the gossips alleged that her change to more natural styling was out of necessity because she had lost so much hair during her pregnancy with the dauphin, it became one of the defining styles of the 1780s in both England and France.

It is very likely that Eliza de Feuillide adopted the style, as she wrote from Paris announcing that she had cut half the length off her hair. Certainly, the scandalous Perdita

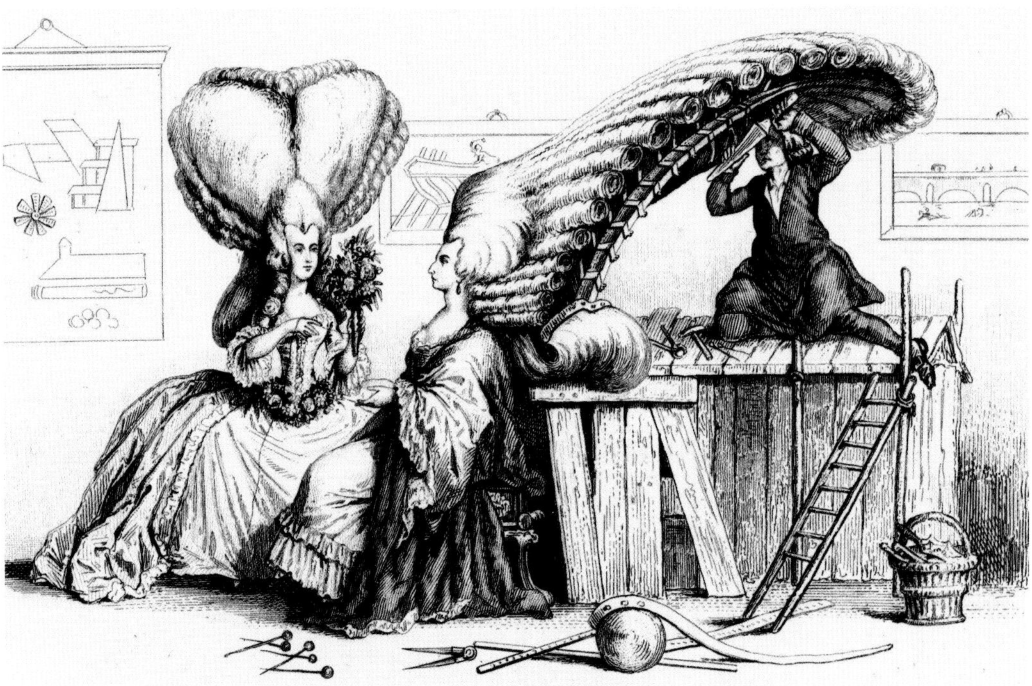

L'Académie pour la coiffures des dames. A satirical drawing of Legros de Rumigny, 'building a head'.

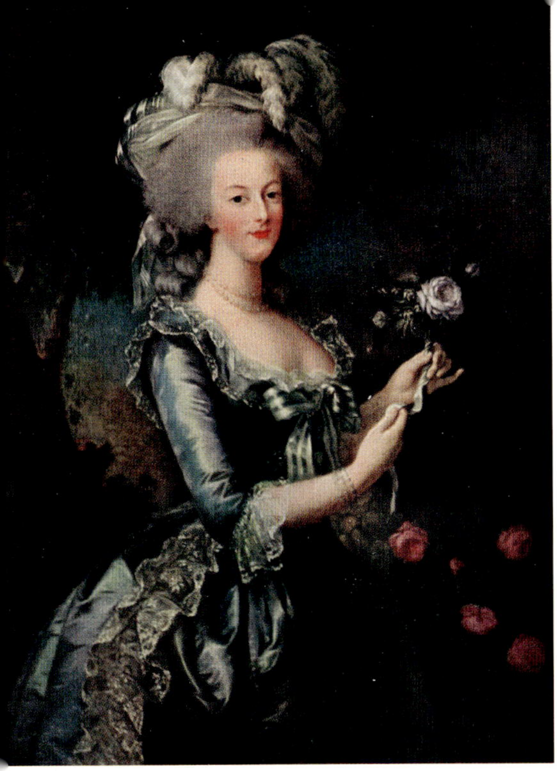

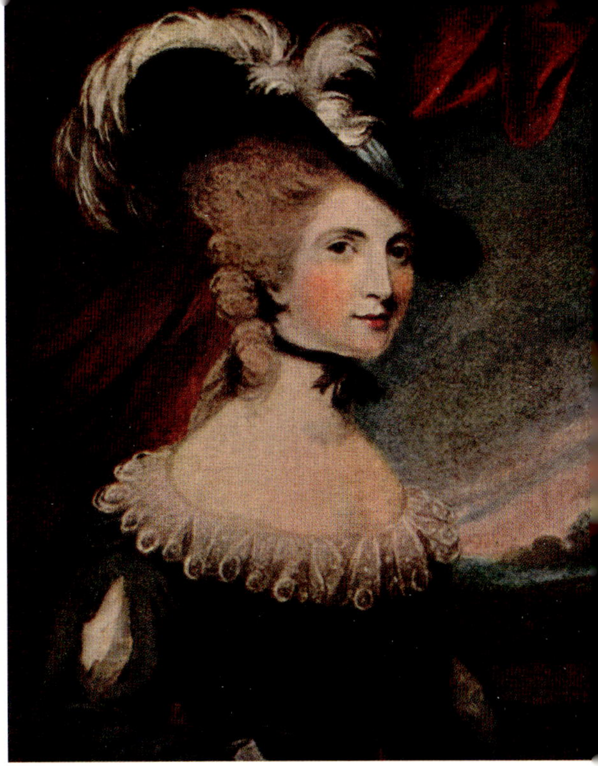

Above left: *Marie Antoinette with a Rose* (Elisabeth Vigée Le Brun, 1783) wearing the influential *Coiffure à l'Enfant*. Ironically, the original portrait – featuring her in a simple muslin gown with a straw hat on her barely powdered hair – was considered too controversial, as a queen should not be seen without her finery.

Above right: *Perdita* (portrait miniature by Charles Bestland). The scandalous actress Perdita Robinson, and lover of the Prince Regent, charmed the French court and became a style icon for her era as everything she wore was immediately copied.

Robinson and Georgiana, Duchess of Devonshire, visited Marie Antoinette at much the same time and returned to England sporting styles very similar to *Coiffure a l'Enfant*, as well as slinky muslin chemise dresses known in France as the *Chemise de la Reine*. Both were pivotal in the change from the rigid styles of the *ancien régime* to the modern, high-waisted silhouette.

As Marie Antoinette wore no *blanc* (white) ceruse, her lovely complexion could only be attributed to her beauty regime of *Eau Cosmetique du Pigeon*, *Eau des Carmes* and *Eau d'Ange*. *Eau des Carmes*, or Carmelite water, had been distilled by the Carmelite monastic order since the sixteenth century and was renowned for the calming and health-giving effects of its lemon balm, angelica and nutmeg. It had been used at the French court since the days of the Sun King as a cordial taken with water or wine to relieve headaches, nervous disorders and minor digestive issues. It could also be used as a toilet water that could be applied to cleanse and revive the complexion (much like modern micellar water), as was the angelic *Eau d'Ange* which was distilled from cloves, cinnamon and coriander seeds sometimes with additional musk to boost its fragrance.

Her *Eau Cosmetique du Pigeon* was also known in Britain as Pigeon's Water, a cosmetic wash concocted to a mysterious recipe and used by the ladies of Denmark, apparently with remarkable results. In a letter to *The Lady's Magazine* in the summer of 1778, the signatory William Wimple asserted: 'Many ladies in this country [Denmark] who are full fifty years of age, preserve by these means all the freshness and bloom of twenty-one.'

Although he stated that the recipe was a closely guarded secret, he revealed that as well as numerous flowers and lemon juice, take:

> Seven or eight white pigeons, pluck them, and cut off the heads and ends of the wings, then mince them very small, and put them, with the other ingredients into an alembic; add also four ounces of double refined sugar, one drachm of borax, and as much camphire; the crumb of four small white loaves new from the oven, and a pint

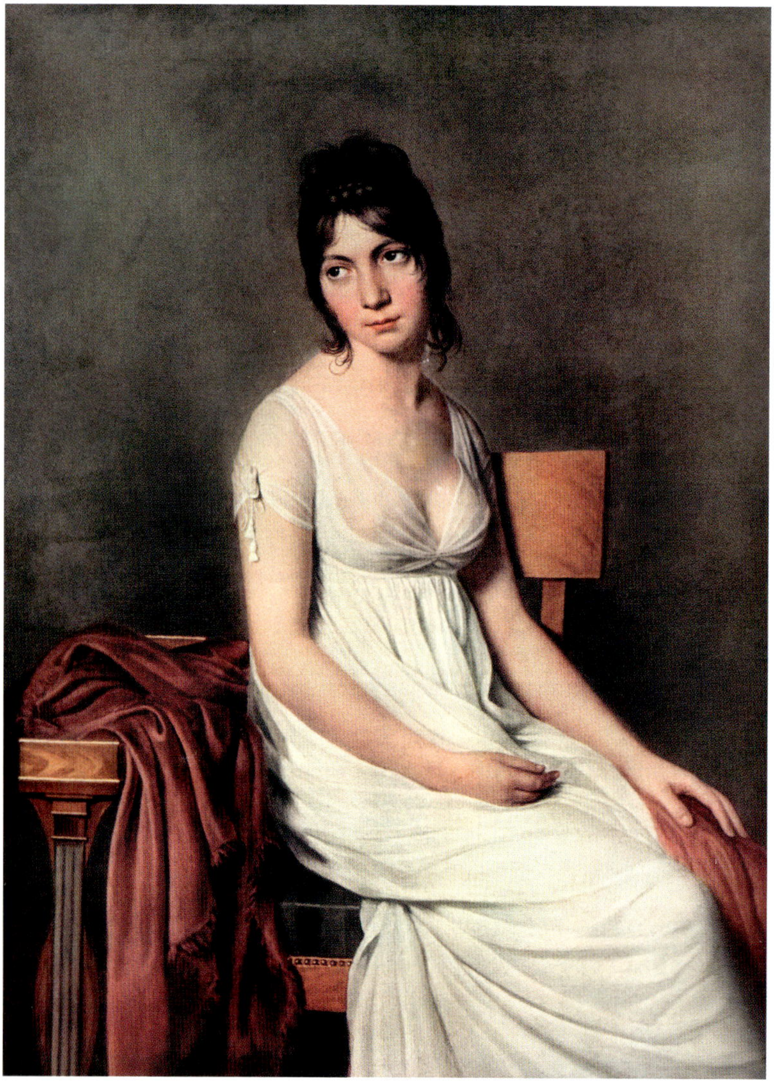

Portrait of a Young Woman in White (Jacques Louis David, 1798). Neoclassical beauty, inspired by Térézia Tallien, she wears cropped hair with a braid of artificial hair and a scant muslin gown sheer across the bosom.

> of good white wine. Let them digest in the alembic seventeen or eighteen days, after which distil the whole and reserve the water for use.

And he finished with the plea: 'This cosmetic I beg leave to recommend to the ladies of Great Britain, instead of those artificial colourings which are now in vogue, and which will inevitably destroy the finest complexion in a short time.'

The writers of the second edition of *The Temple of Flora* (published in 1784) were certainly delighted to accept Wimple's recommendation and included an almost identical version of his recipe.

In 1793, during the years of 'The Terror', the 'Law of Suspects' created Revolutionary Tribunals where anyone considered to be less than supportive of the Republic was dealt with summary mob justice. Aristocrats who couldn't manage to flee to England or Germany went into hiding, stripped bare of their finery as anyone with even a hint of aristocratic style, any make-up or even a whiff of perfume was accused of being counter-revolutionary and sent to the guillotine for their 'crimes' of cosmetics. Jane's cousin Eliza was in England when she heard that her husband, the Count de Feuillide, had met *la guillotine* in February 1794, news that would make the horror of the Revolution shockingly real to all of the Austen family.

Determined to eradicate all signifiers of the *ancien régime*, when the revolutionaries came to execute Marie Antoinette, the first thing they did was hack off her legendary hair. The Princess de Lamballe had been renowned for her beautiful white complexion, so when she was murdered as part of the Revolutionary Tribunal September Massacres of 1793, her body was stripped, mutilated and left naked in the street for all to see her beautiful white skin, a supposed hallmark of the corrupt the *ancien régime*.

Such was the fear of beauty and feminine wiles that when revolutionary leader Robespierre arrested Térézia Tallien and hauled her before a Revolutionary Tribunal the following year she was found to be a counter-revolutionary, guilty of criminal seduction. Térézia was condemned to the guillotine, with Robespierre's personal additional stipulation that she must be held in solitary confinement – presumably so she could not enchant anyone else with her beauty.

Her captors stripped her naked to view her entrancing 'goddess-like' figure and hacked off her towering chignon of jet-black hair, leaving her with nothing more than a dirty chemise. She spent twenty-five days alone in the filthy dungeon whilst her lover organised the coup that deposed and executed Robespierre and ended the Terror. Ironically, just as Robespierre had feared, Térézia was credited with instigating the counter-revolution, having inspired Tallien with the power of her beauty.

She emerged from her cell the darling of Europe. She had nothing more than the scant chemise tied below the bosom with a handkerchief – not even her hair. But in her humiliation, she had redesigned and reclaimed fashion. Such was her heroism the aristocratic survivors finally felt they could re-emerge, and in a flood of joy they reclaimed Paris.

Le Bal des Victimes did much to reunite what was left of the aristocracy. Only those who had lost immediate family to the guillotine were admissible. In grim acknowledgement of their mourning, both men and women wore their hair *à la victime* where the hair was shaven from the back of the neck, then the rest cropped and brought forward in a tousled fringe. Many ladies completed the statement with a narrow scarlet ribbon around their throats as a tribute to their family members who had known Madame Guillotine.

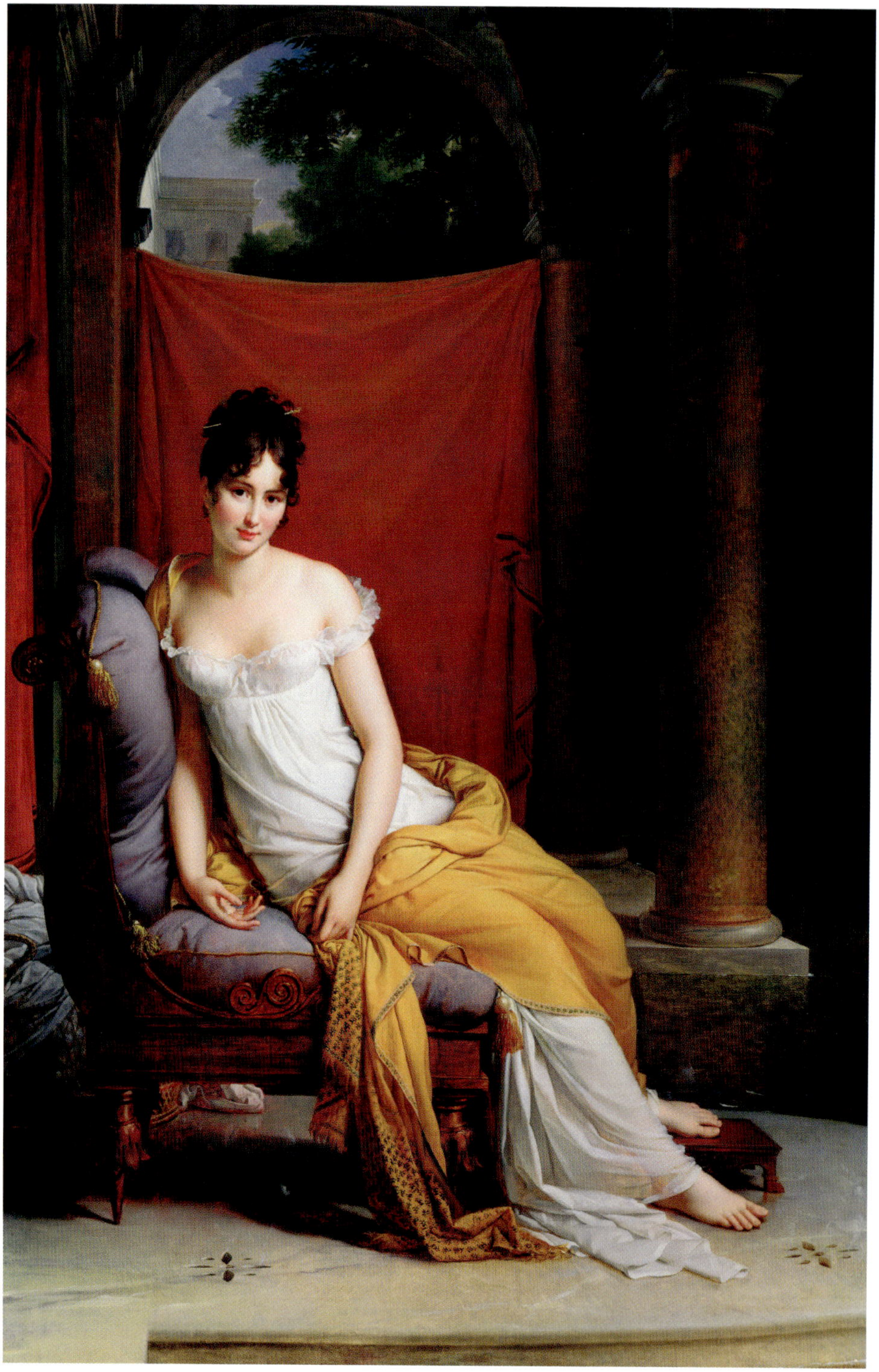

Madame Juliette Recamier (François Gérard, *c.* 1800). When she visited London in March 1802, she was mobbed by people desperate to gaze upon her legendary beauty and it was reported that 'praise poetry and applause follow her everywhere she goes'.

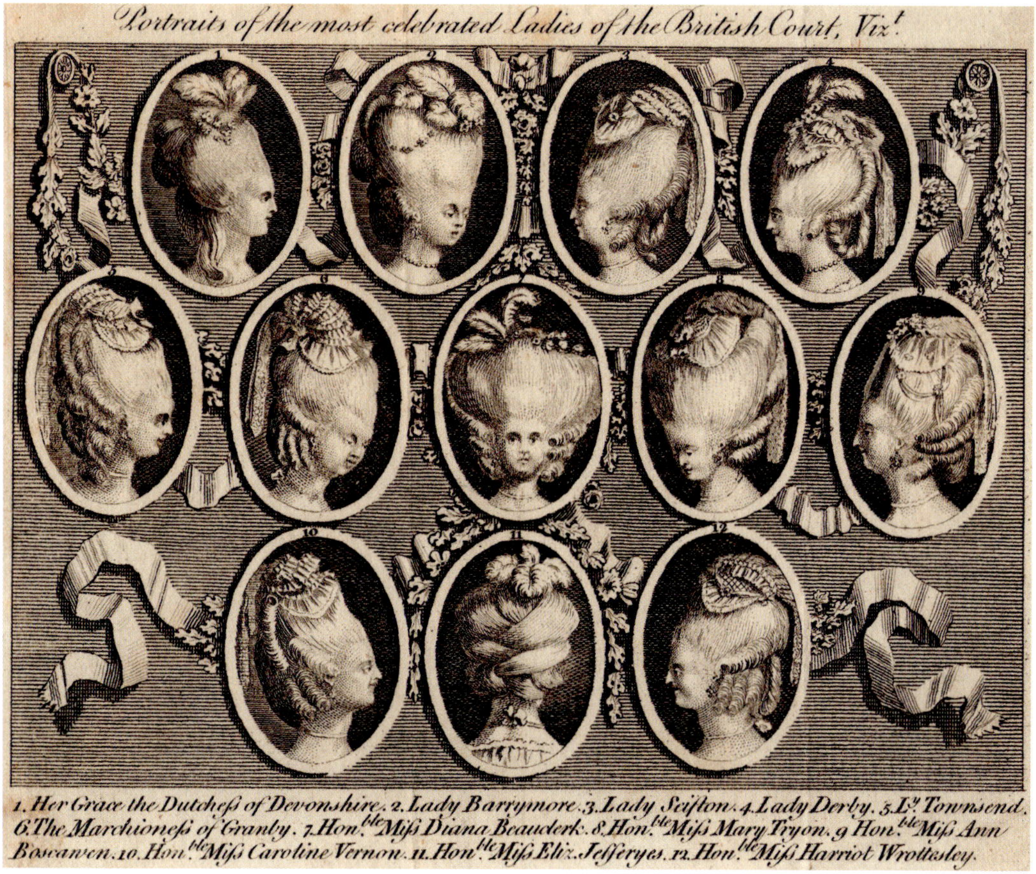

Portraits of the most celebrated ladies of the British court (contemporary magazine *c.* 1780). They loved the traditional towering formal styles and were reluctant to abandon them.

appearance of the eyes and face', and for those with red hair 'a deep brown or chocolate powder gives the happiest cast'.

In 1782, London hairdresser James Stewart published *Plocacosmos: or the Whole Art of Hairdressing; wherein is contained Ample Rules for the Young Artizan, more particularly for Ladies, Women, Valets, etc. etc. as well as directions for Persons to dress their own Hair, also Ample and Wholesome Rules to preserve the Hair.* Stewart insists that the fat of 'a young and healthy animal' should be used as the basis for pomatum, especially calves, hogs and bears, but adds that eel's fat is also 'esteemed to take away the pits of the small pox and to make the hair grow'. Notwithstanding this, it was the grease of that most hirsute of creatures, the brown bear, that became renowned in Regency England as the most effective for promoting hair growth and restoring the beauty of the hair. Legend has it that Atkinson's Bear's Grease Pomade – reputedly used by Beau Brummel, Lady Emma Hamilton and the Duke of Wellington – originated in 1799 when the founder James Atkinson made the long journey from Cumberland to London on foot. He had walked with his (presumably tame) bear, but upon arrival at his shop in Gerrard Street

2

A Tax on Beauty or Attacks on Beauty

Britain's beauties had always taken their inspiration from the glamorous standards of the French court, but the radical changes during the Revolutionary years were not so easy to embrace. As one of London's first celebrity hairdressers, William Barker, notes in his *Treatise on the Principles of Hair-Dressing; in which the Deformities of Modern Hairdressing are pointed out, and an elegant and natural Plan recommended, upon Hogarth's immortal System of Beauty*: 'Strange, that no sooner had the French queen discarded the "absurd" mode of hair-dressing than the English ladies now adhere to the ridiculous mode which the Queen is endeavouring to abolish.'

English ladies, especially those of the court of George III, were clinging on to traditional styles and beauty techniques as well as the noble status bestowed by them. This elegant throwback position was compounded by the steady trickle of deposed French aristocrats who wanted nothing more than to take refuge in an elegant haven within the safe order of the past.

Inspired by Georgiana of Devonshire and Perdita Robinson, many women transitioned to softer styles with curls flowing about their shoulders and less height, albeit still formed with powder and pomatum. Dressing the hair with pomatum and powder not only thickened and boosted thinning hair, these products added height and volume, helped set the hair in curl and in place, and were also very effective in concealing thinning hair and blending in any artificial tresses that might be added. Grey roots could also be effectively blended in by mixing a little ivory black artist's pigment into white pomatum and carefully brushing it into the roots with a small brush; once powdered over, it was difficult to distinguish a difference from natural dark hair.

With its lovely warm-brown tint, Mareschal hair powder coloured with ground cinnamon and cloves became very popular, not least for its scent. William Barker advocated a move away from traditional pure-white powder to create a more natural look which tastefully complimented the skin and hair tones of the individual. Certainly, for more natural complexions without any heavy white make-up, the contrast of white hair powder could give an unflattering tint to the complexion so a little brown tint could 'enliven the

Right: *A Lady in a Brown Dress: 'The Parson's Daughter'* (George Romney, 1785). Her hair is based on the *Coiffure à l'Enfant* and powdered with tinted Mareschal hair powder.

Below left: Georgiana, Duchess of Devonshire (Thomas Gainsborough, 1783). Both widely admired and emulated, she and Perdita were in perpetual rivalry to be leaders of fashion.

Below right: An illustration from *Plocacosmos: Or the Whole Art of Hairdressing* (1782) depicting perfectly craped and frizzed hair based on the *Coiffure à l'Enfant*, sometimes known as 'the Hedgehog'.

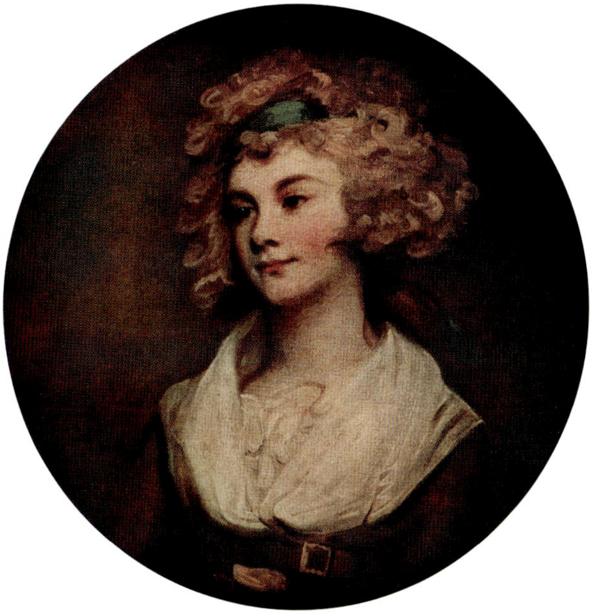

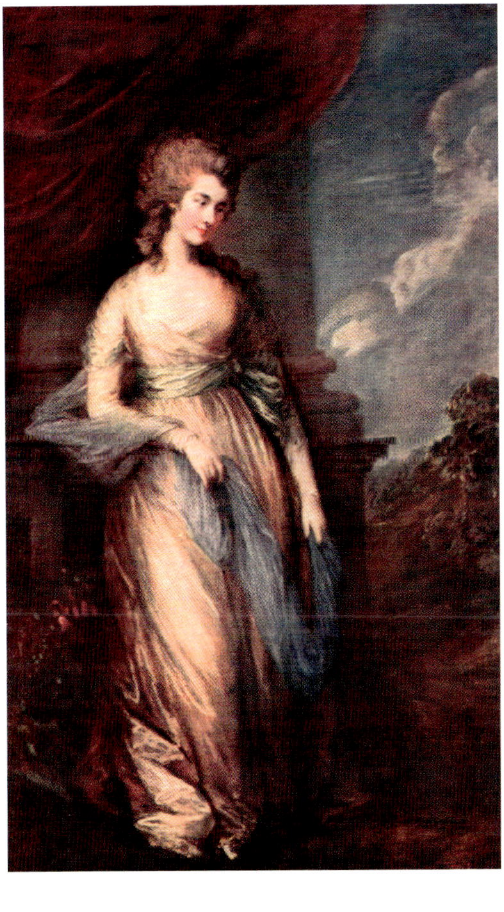

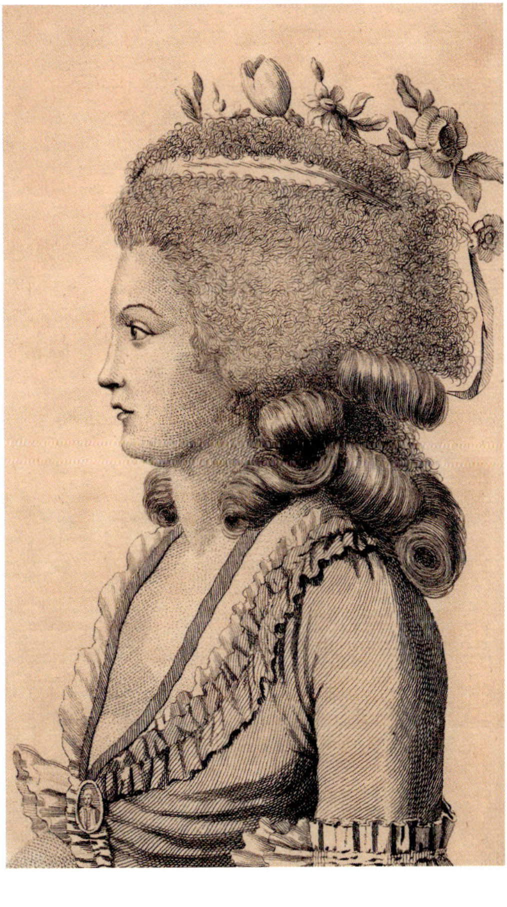

he tied it up outside to advertise his bear's grease before sacrificing the poor creature to make the celebrated hair care product.

Frizzing and craping were the techniques used to add height and volume to the hair. In *Plocacosmos,* James Stewart gives a characteristically detailed and lengthy description of the process: first, smoothing the hair with hard pomade that contained wax as well as fat and then twisting the hair until it curls in a ball tight to the head: 'When all is done, they look like regular rows of trees, truly set, with their heads bending to the crown, as if blown thence by a gust of wind from the face.' Each is then wrapped in a curling paper and heated with the curling tongs until it smoked. Pomatum was useful to smooth the ends of hair when wrapping curling papers to set curls, but application to the roots must be avoided as the oil would burn the scalp when heat was applied. Once cooled and the paper removed, it would be carefully unwrapped to avoid knotting and then back-combed firmly to create volume at the roots whilst retaining its original length. This voluminous frizz could then be teased and sculpted into the required shape, which would last very well with only a weekly touch up of fresh pomade and powder applied.

Hair powder had to be of the best quality with no adulteration, particularly from lime or plaster, as this could result in the scalp becoming raised in a painful, hot rash with the hair

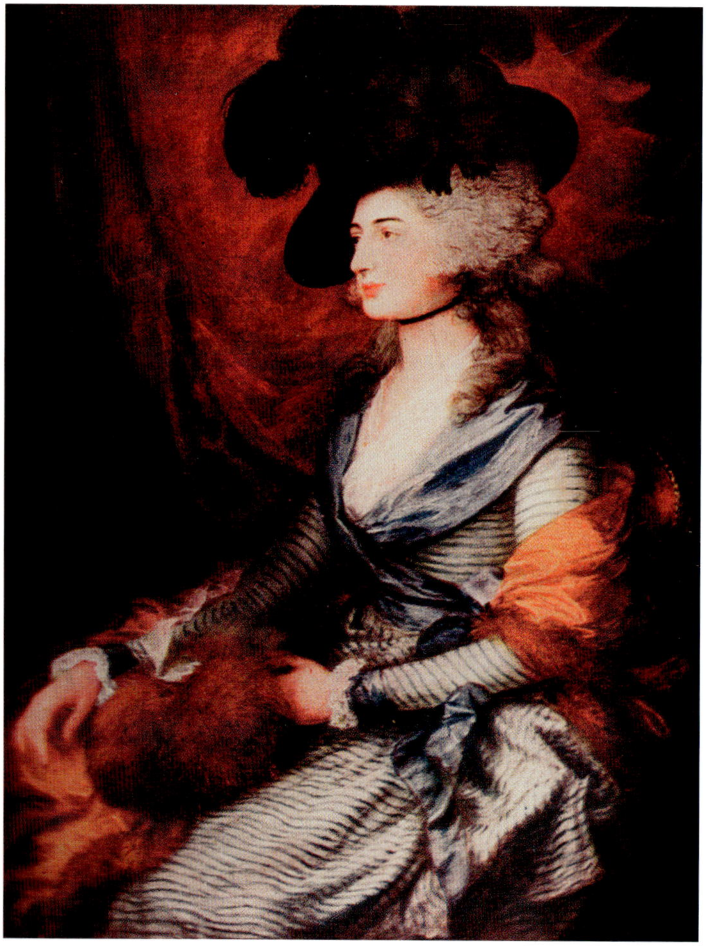

Left: Sarah Siddons (Thomas Gainsborough, 1785). William Barker has artfully frizzled her hair to complement her features, and the high ribbon choker compliments her elegant neck.

Opposite: *La Toilette D'un Clerc De Procureur* (Philibert Louis Debucourt, 1816). The gentleman wears a powder gown to protect his clothes and a cone shape mask to cover his face as the hairdresser wafts copious amounts of hair powder from his powder bag.

breaking off at the root. It had to be applied with a good-quality swansdown puff. The final touch once the style was fully created was to fill a wig bellows with hair powder and gently puff a fine smoke of powder into the roots of the hair, which would allow for full coverage without excess on the surface. Any drifts of powder that had gathered at the hairline could be gently removed with a blunt powder knife.

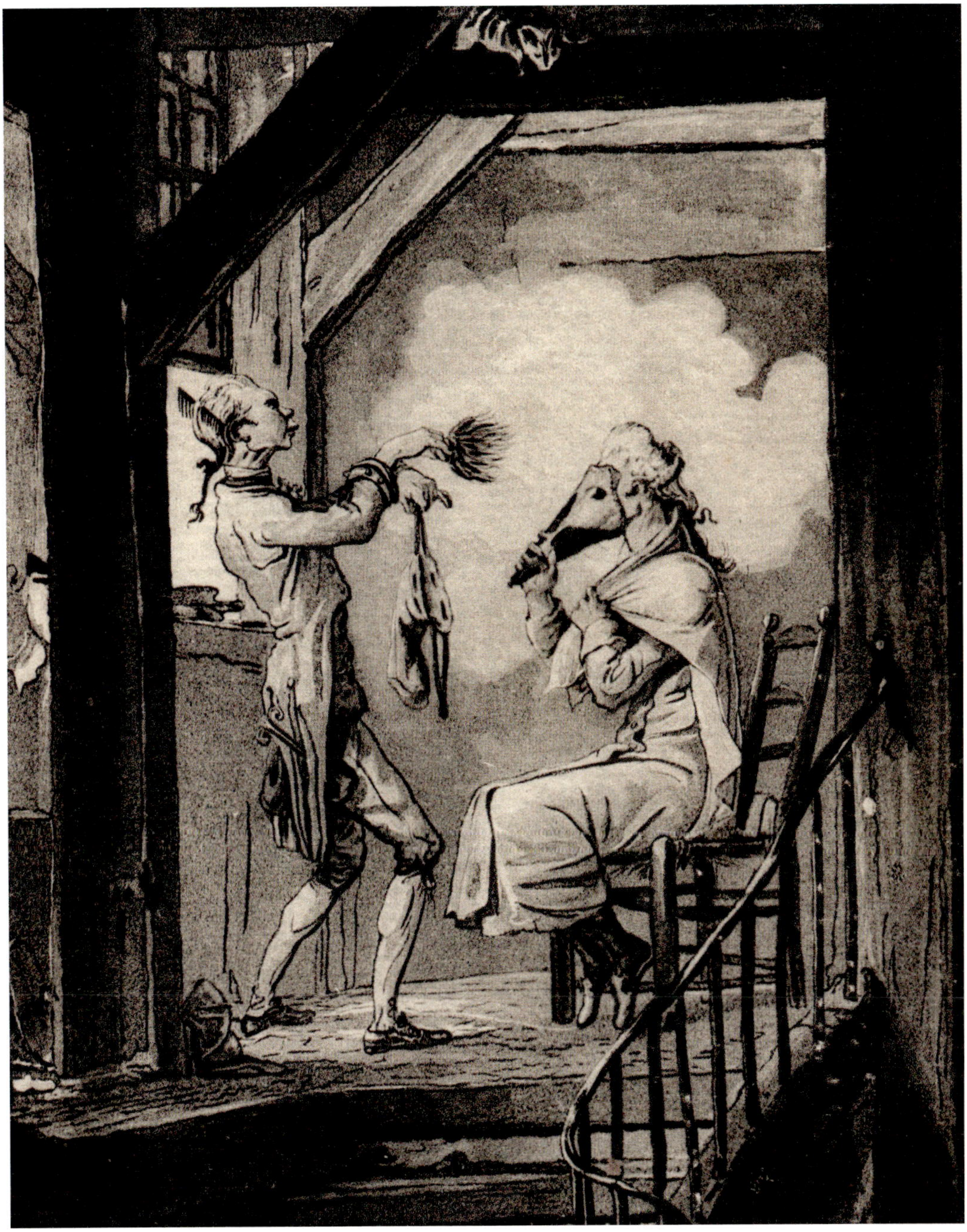

Wigs would be sent out to a hairdresser or barber to be powdered, but inevitably with use of such large quantities of powder, it would get everywhere. Fashionable households would have a dedicated powder room or powder closet off the dressing room to minimise fall out. Within, there would be a powder gown or a large cloth to protect the clothes during the final powdering, as well as a conical mask that would protect the face whilst being powdered and a selection of stands for wigs and hair pieces.

However, in 1795 hair powder was to become political. Prime Minister William Pitt had already introduced a plethora of taxes to fund the wars, but as the Revolutionary Wars dragged into the Napoleonic Wars it became imperative to raise more money. Quite a significant portion of the population had become accustomed to using hair powder – those of the aristocratic and genteel classes as well as the clergy, the armed forces, not to mention almost everyone's servants – so there was potentially plenty of tax revenue to be gained by charging a guinea for an annual licence. In an attempt to make the tax slightly more acceptable Pitt made some exceptions: members of the clergy (like Jane Austen's father) with a low income; members of the armed forces, who had to have powdered hair for uniform dress; and gentlemen like Mr Bennet with more than two unmarried daughters could purchase licences for two and receive licences for the other daughters for free.

Many felt it was a tax too far and, in a faint echo of the French counter-Revolutionary protest of the coiffure *à la victime*, they cropped their hair to oppose the tax. The satirists

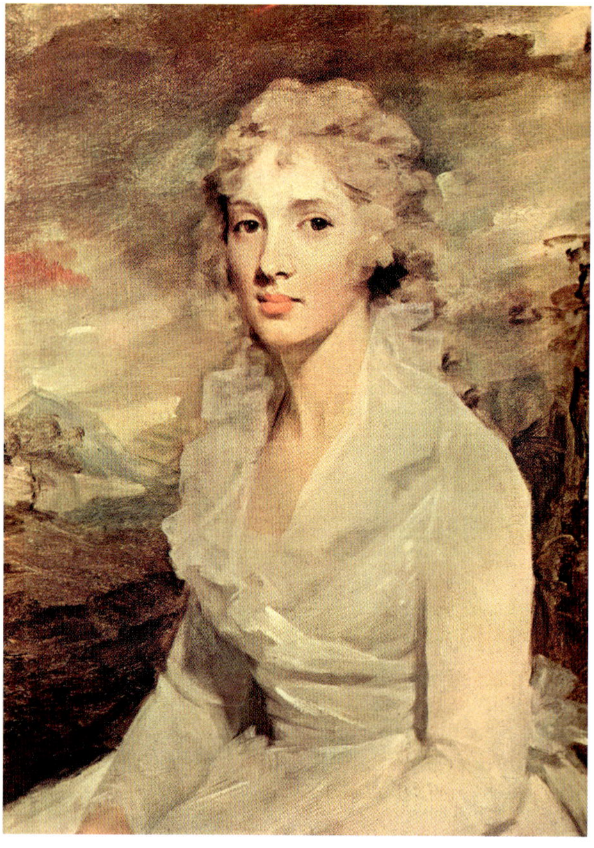

Miss Eleanor Urquhart (Sir Henry Raeburn, 1793). During the 1790s frizzled styles softened into a more natural tumble of loose curls that didn't necessarily require powder and pomatum.

dubbed the conformists as 'Guinea Pigs', as the tax cost a guinea per annum, and the deposers as the 'Crop Club'.

There was already a decline in the use of hair powder as frizzed and craped styles softened into curls, but magazines such as Heideloff's *Gallery of Fashion* continued to show powdered styles until 1803. Nevertheless, the tax had a polarising effect, with traditionalists claiming that after a century of powdering it was indecent to go without. The army renounced its use in 1799, and as the century reached its final years of crop failures, rising prices and corn riots, a head powdered even with the inedible part of the wheat crop made a profound statement in the face of severe hunger.

Fashion was always a popular subject for the critical gaze of satirists like Thomas Rowlandson and James Gillray, but in the 1790s with such radical changes in silhouette and style, they were able to attack from both sides, mocking both the absurdity and tastelessness of those quick to embrace the new and also the pitiful old dames who could not – or would not – move with the times. For, as ever, it was women who bore the brunt of the criticism.

Accusations of women being poor and neglectful mothers were popular and had a frisson of moral outrage, as did insinuations of infidelity, but nothing was as much fun as the shrieks of 'mutton dressed as lamb', shaming women for their attempts to improve their looks.

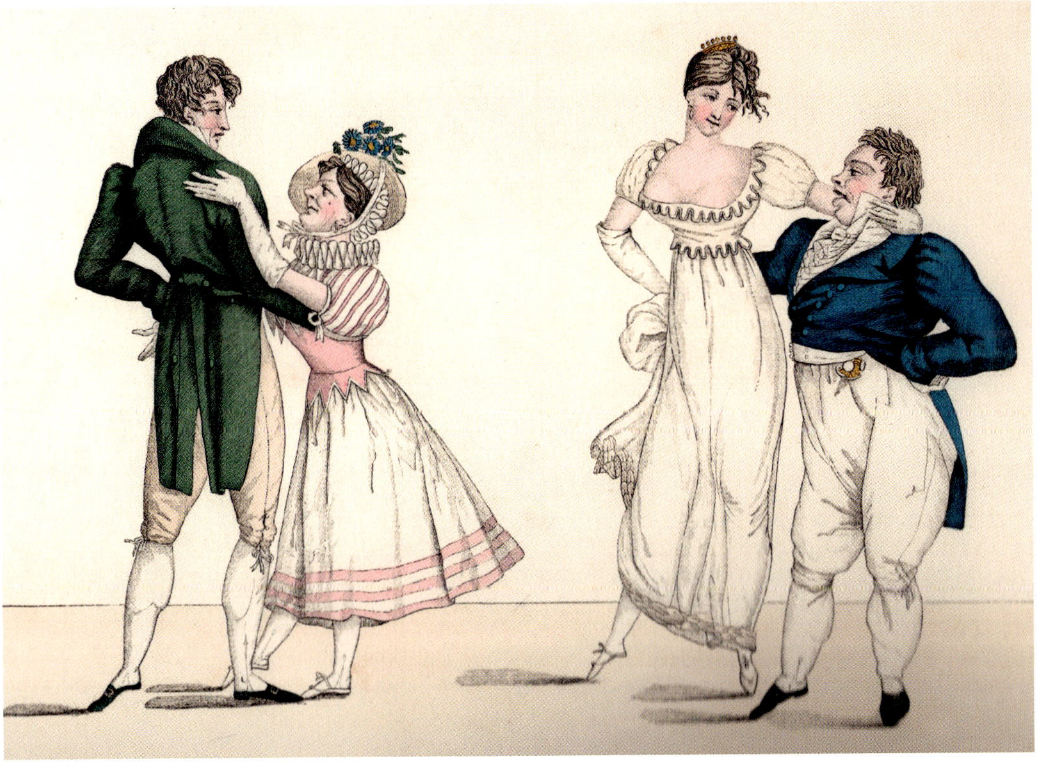

Les Contrastes (Le Bon Genre, 1806). Those of short stature were also considered fair game by satirists on both sides of the Channel.

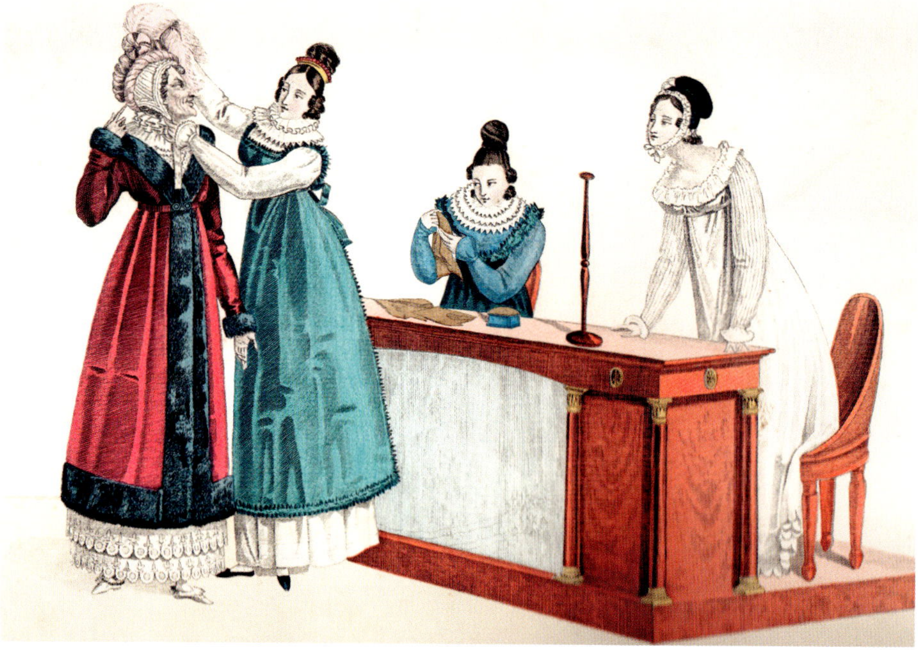

Le Contraste au Chapeau Coleur de Rose (Le Bon Genre, 1815). There was much criticism of older women wearing 'young' fashions, particularly anything in pink.

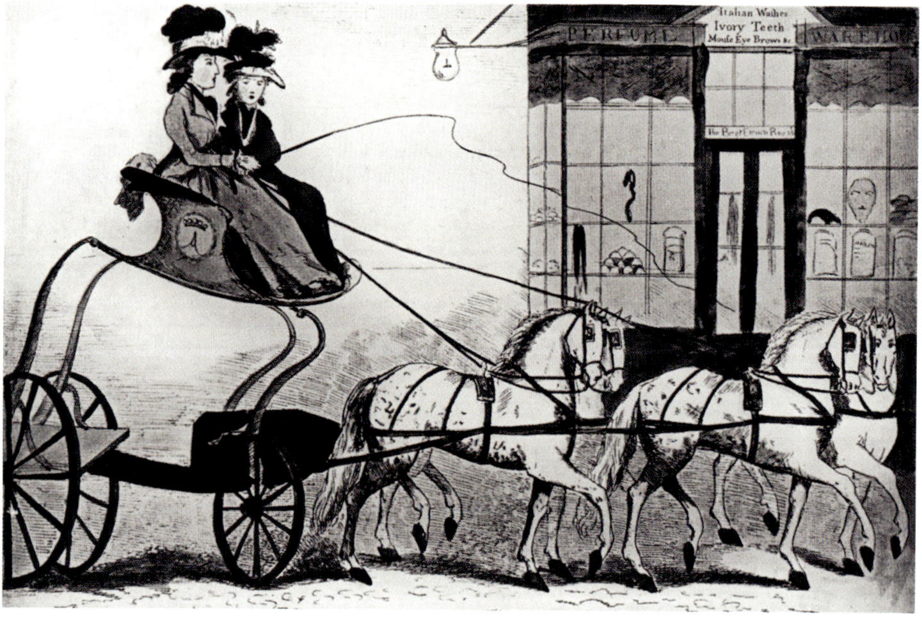

'The Portland Place A--R Driving Without a Beau to R---D's Perfume Warehouse' (C. Clark, June 1782). A caricature of Lady Sarah Archer dashing at high speed to buy more cosmetics at the Perfume Warehouse, which boasts a stock of: 'Italian Washes, Mouse Eye Brows, Ivory Teeth, artificial tresses and *Bezt French Roush*'.

With so many men away at war, women were more visible and as they began to make inroads in art, culture and, with the first anti-slavery boycotts, politics, the satirists began to sharpen their pencils and their knives. Lady Sarah Archer was popular game; she was the daughter of a prominent politician and the wealthy widow of a Warwickshire baron with four teenage daughters. The satirists were relentless, castigating her as a bad mother, accusing her of selfishly trying to prevent her daughters from marrying, caricaturing her abilities as a fine 'whip' and attacking her for her gambling prowess, but most of all they attacked her for her looks and use of cosmetics. Depicted as a crone with a large, hooked nose and bright vermillion-encrusted cheeks, she was parodied as a painted harridan. Jane's friend, the author Fanny Burney, had met Lady Archer and commented on her absurdly high headdress. She also noted that when Lady Archer was viewed at close range her complexion was a 'most unnatural cake of white and red'.

The most brutal attack came in 1792 from Thomas Rowlandson with 'Six Stages of Mending a Face – Dedicated with respect to the Right Hon.ble Lady Sarah Archer', which draws upon the catalogue of extreme artifice and repulsive beauty aids listed in Jonathan Swift's poem 'A Beautiful Young Nymph Going To Bed' (1731) that suggest that a woman's beauty routine – especially that of an older woman who would inevitably be in need of

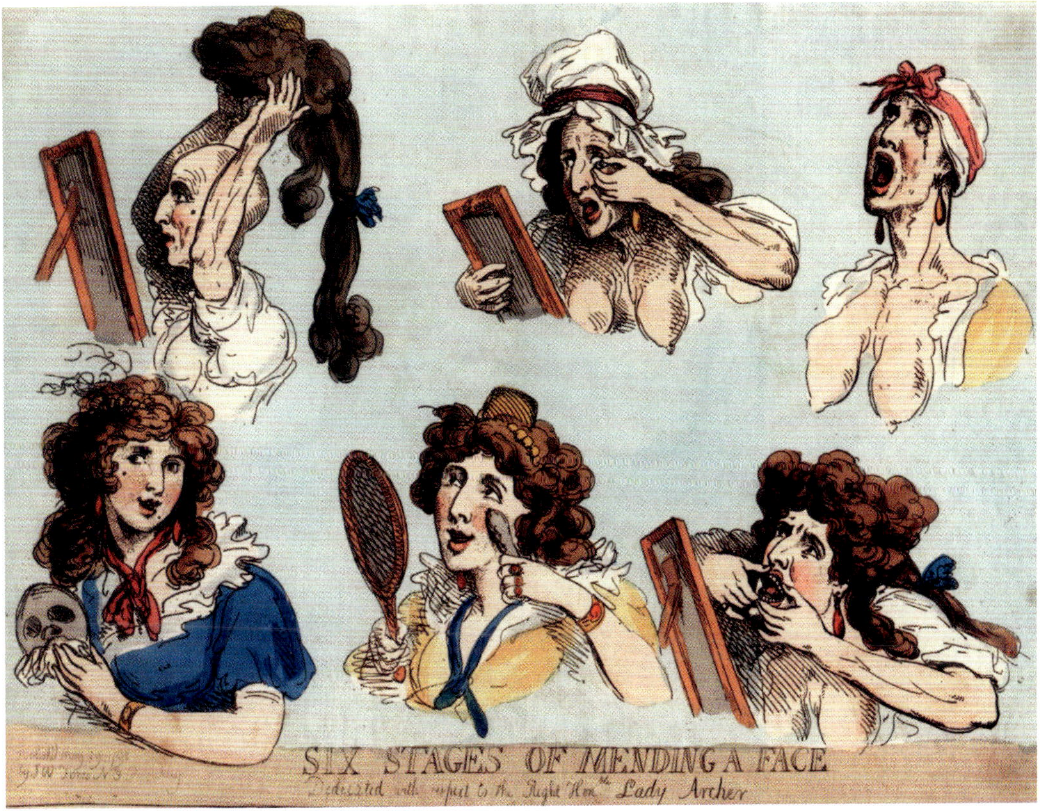

'Six Stages of Mending a Face – Dedicated with Respect to the Right Hon.ble Lady Sarah Archer' (Thomas Rowlandson, 1792).

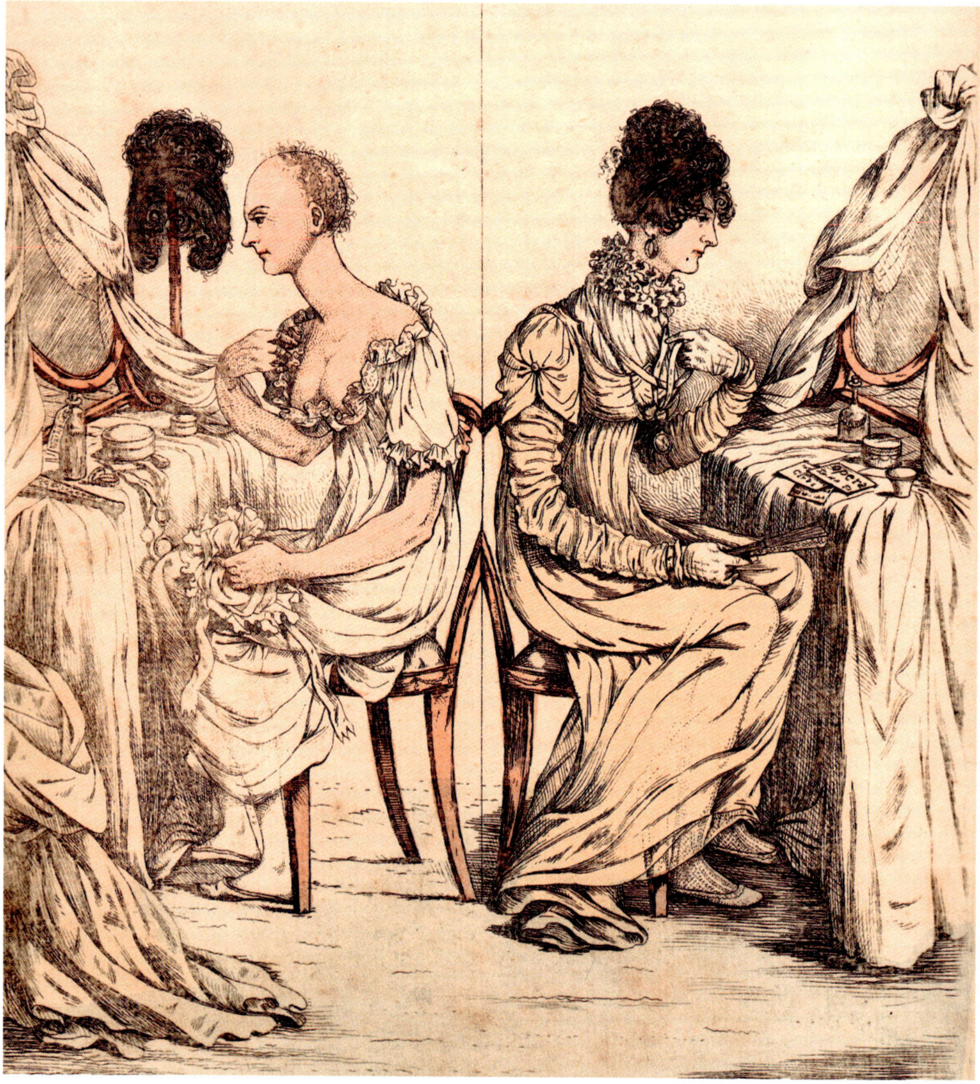

'A Fashionable Lady in Dress and Undress' (Robert Dighton, 1807). Another satire to reveal that a beautiful woman might be no more than the sum of her artificial parts.

extensive regeneration – was a foetid and revolting affair. The 'six stages' depicted are a wig to cover her baldness, a glass eye, artificial teeth, 'plumpers' (the balls of cork or fabric used to pad out hollow, toothless cheeks), rouge applied with a hare's foot, and padding to support her bosom. In the final illustration she looks pretty and stylish, but she is holding a mask representative of the masquerade.

There was also the deep-seated misogynistic Freudian fear about women's private spaces and what happened within. Jonathan Swift's poem 'The Lady's Dressing Room' (1730) gives the tale of haughty Celia, who after spending five hours about her toilette emerges looking like a goddess, but her servant, who sneaks into her dressing room to survey the litter she has left behind, is repulsed by what he finds: her dirty smock and soiled stockings, smelly towels and dirty combs full of 'sweat, dandruff, powder, lead, and hair'. She also reportedly has 'pomatums, paints and slops, and ointments good for scabby chops'.

Conversely, there were also concerns about older women being too attractive and desirable. As this age of wars progressed, taking almost a third of British men of fighting age, the number of widows quickly multiplied and without husbands to police their behaviour this group of women might do anything! There was a deep-seated fear of the mature woman who could take pleasure freely without fear of pregnancy.

The idea that older women might steal focus from the debutantes seeking husbands from an already much-depleted stock was appalling. As one young lady wrote to *The Lady's Monthly Museum* in December 1800:

> SIR,
> I AM a very pretty girl, and not above sixteen. I am universally admired – nay, followed, and even made a fuss with – and yet, would you believe it, I have not a lover in my train! After having examined my whole person in my glass several times, without discovering any faults, I began to imagine that there was something in my dress to render it forbidding. Determined, therefore, to make some regulations in it, I sent for a new hair-dresser, and a new mantua-maker; but I could not gain my point with all my endeavours. My patience being at last quite exhausted, I ventured to ask a smart fellow, one night, at Ranelagh, on his comparing me to an angel, what he meant?

He explained that although he found her beautiful, 'married women, child, are the only women in the world to flirt with; for who, in his sober senses, would chuse, in these ticklish and expensive times, to have a wife of his own?' The letter continues:

> You cannot conceive, Sir, how much I was mortified by this answer. Government, surely, ought to put a stop, by some speedy methods, to the proceedings of the married women in this licentious age, who engross the men to themselves, and hinder us poor girls from getting husbands.
>
> I am Sir, your very humble servant,
> (in spite of all my disappointments)
> FANNY FORWARD

The satirists' favourite topic for hilarity by far was how pathetic it was when a pitiful, ugly, old, scrawny woman persisted in trying to be pretty. The cruelty levied against those who had aged beyond thirty and been 'left on the shelf' knew no bounds. In *Emma*, Jane Austen describes Miss Bates as 'neither young, handsome, rich, nor married' with 'neither beauty or cleverness' and with 'no intellectual superiority'. However, to her credit, she likes everyone and she has a 'contented temper'. Emma says: 'A single woman, with a very narrow income, must be a ridiculous, disagreeable, old maid ... but a single woman, of good fortune, is always respectable, and may be as sensible and pleasant as anybody else.'

With Miss Bates, Jane makes it painfully clear just how much was at stake if you failed to win a husband. This was a sentiment echoed by Jane's contemporary Maria Edgeworth,

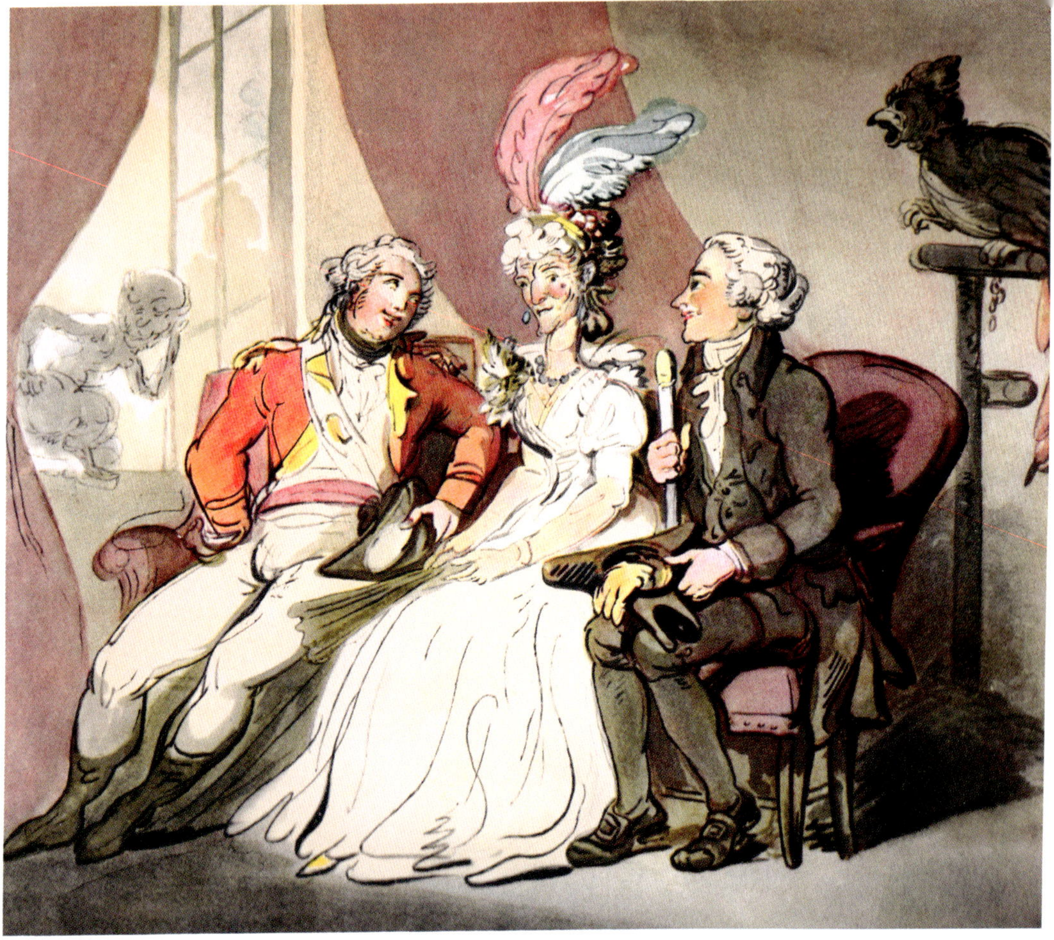

The Rivals (Thomas Rowlandson, 1786). Two younger men competing for the hand – or rather the wealth – of an elderly spinster because the law decreed that from the moment she married her possessions became those of her husband.

the author of *Belinda,* who wrote in her *Letters for Literary Ladies* (1795) that she admired the 'good sense' of the 'celebrated modern beauty' who wished 'that she might not survive her nine-and-twentieth birthday' because she 'foresaw the inevitable doom of her declining years. Her apprehensions for the future embittered even her enjoyment of the present; and she had resolution enough to offer to take "a bond of fate," to sacrifice one half of her life, to secure the pleasure of the other.'

3

Beauty in Hiding

With the Industrial Revolution and the birth of magazine culture, horizons expanded exponentially. Where once an apothecary had made products only for his shop and clientele of trade professional and retail purchasers, the ability to manufacture a product, create a brand, package it and advertise it throughout the nation to a market of interested consumers was a revelation. It would be interesting to know if Eliza de Feuillide used

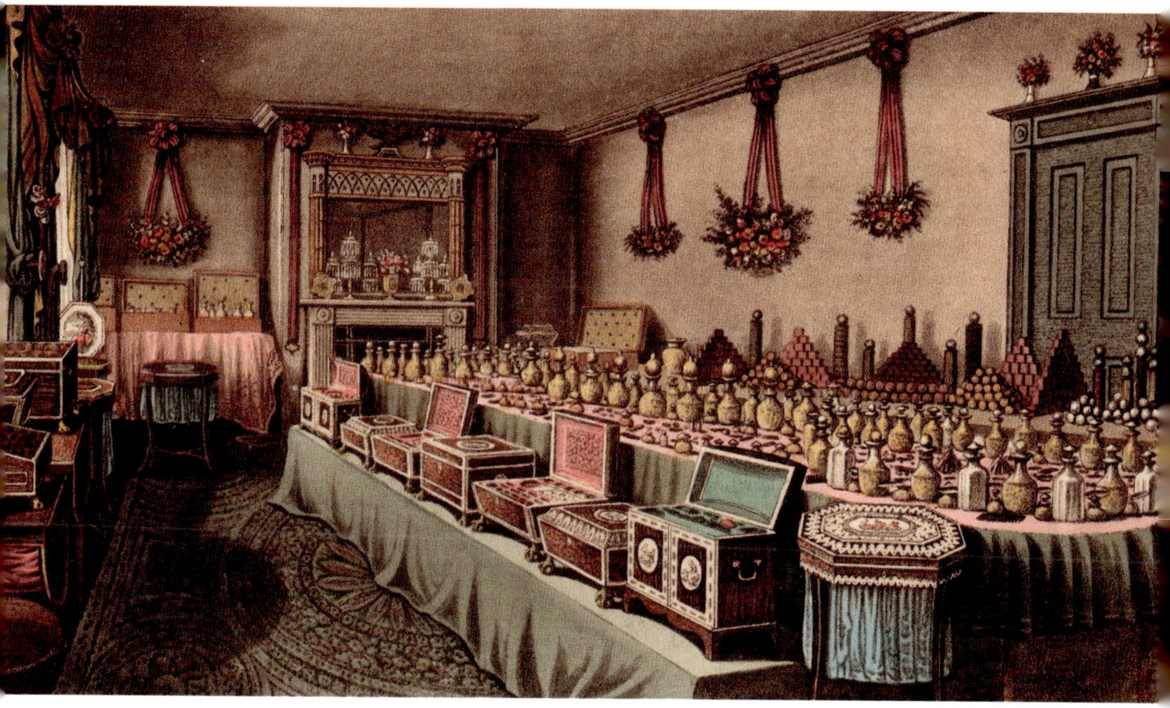

Mr Ross's Room, Bishopsgate Street, a perfumery so renowned for its beautiful displays of perfume and cosmetics that it was featured as a notable London destination in Ackermann's *Repository of Arts* in 1816.

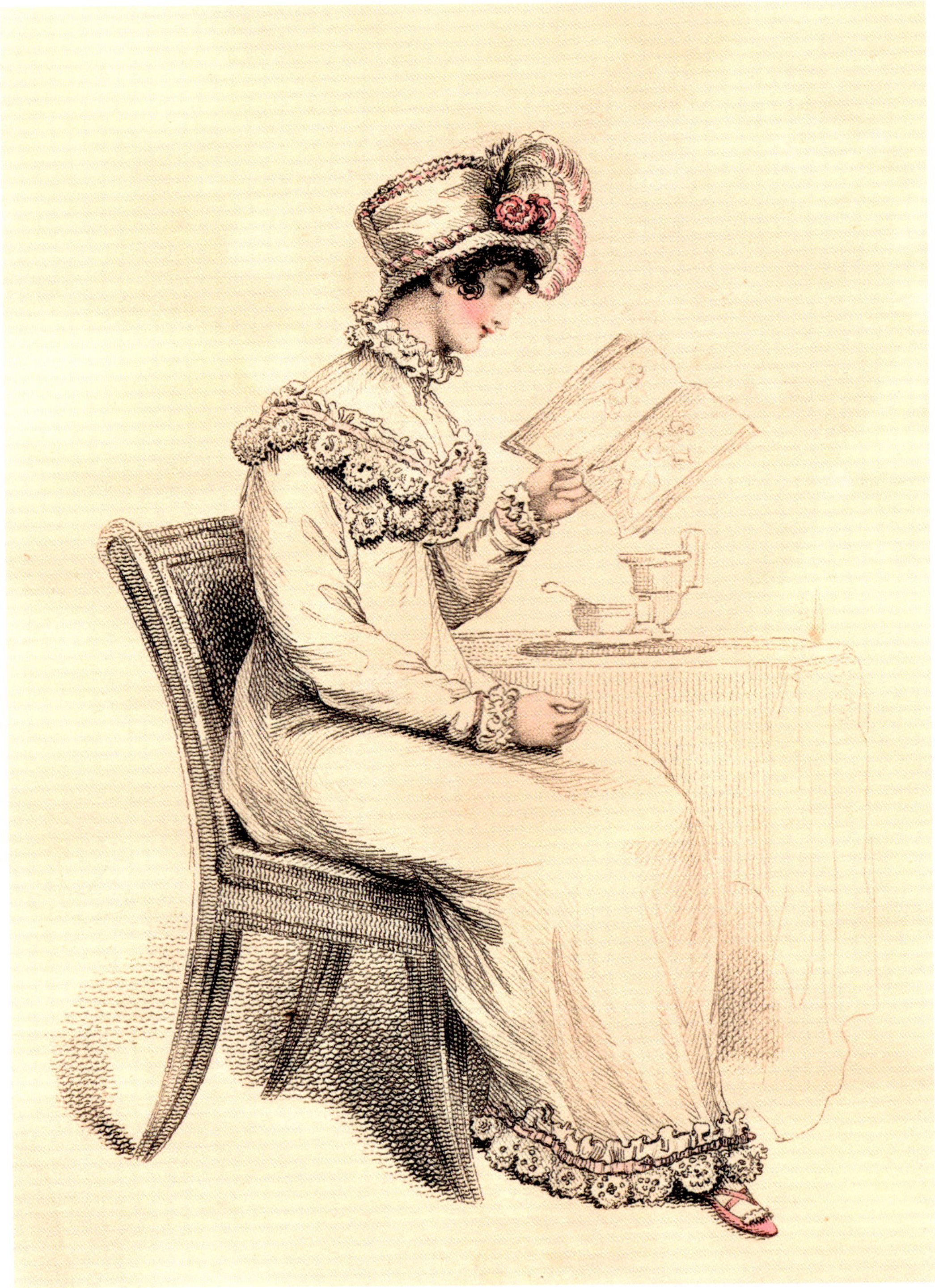

'Morning Dress', *La Belle Assemblée*, July 1815. The birth of magazine culture brought new style inspiration each month, as well as advertising to promote access to the new generation of commercially available beauty products.

Olympian Dew, as it was one of the first products commercially available and one of the most celebrated. An advert from 1784 proclaimed that Marie Antoinette used it:

> To the ladies Olympian Dew, or Crecian bloom water, is recommended, being the only thing discovered that will effectually clear the skin ... it instantly makes wrinkles disappear, and gives a loveliness to the countenance too charming to be described. This elegant article is not only used all over Europe as a cosmetic by the ladies (and by gentlemen after shaving) ... [there is] No perfume so sweet, so delicate, so refreshing, as Olympian Dew, says the Queen of France; she not only uses it herself, but has commanded all her attendant Nobility to do the same.

There was an enormous pressure on the Regency belle; her face was her fortune, the only card she had to play in the high stakes game of matrimony. She had always had to be beautiful, graceful, elegant and charming, but in the age of Rousseau she now also had to be natural. This was all very well for the tiny percentage blessed at birth with the genes for thick, lustrous hair, limpid eyes beautifully framed with long eyelashes and well-formed eyebrows (like Jane Fairfax) and a perfect, clear complexion, as well as the facial symmetry that universally appeals. However, for those gifted with problem hair, pale, insipid features and teenage acne, being a 'natural' beauty could take a lot of work!

With growing awareness of the problems resulting from the use of poisonous lead and mercury-based make-up, advertisers resorted to euphemistic claims for their 'natural' products. Items for the complexion were certainly not 'paints', only 'washes' to cleanse and revive the skin, and rouge was simply a little bloom to restore the natural roses that should rightfully be in the cheeks. It was definitely not an artificial enhancement, only a health or beauty problem being identified and resolved.

However, while this paradigm shift away from a woman being creative with her beauty to one where she had problems and deficiencies might have legitimised the use of aids to restore natural beauty, it also legitimised a cultural standpoint where a woman was to be viewed and assessed for her flaws, and a man was to be paid for a product to resolve them.

As beauty was reframed as natural, it inevitably became 'young' and 'wrinkle free'; the signs of aging were almost as frightening to Regency beauty standards as they are to us today. It was as if women should be ashamed of aging, especially beyond the age of thirty, which was regarded as the gateway to old age. Even Jane comments in a letter of 9 December 1808, a few days shy of her thirty-third birthday:

> Our ball was rather more amusing than I expected ... It was the same room in which we danced fifteen years ago! I thought it all over, and in spite of the shame of being so much older, felt with thankfulness that I was quite as happy now as then.

In *Persuasion*, written in 1815–16 when she reached forty, Jane explores aging as an aspect of the story of Anne Elliot and her lost love. She is the least favourite of Sir Walter's daughters, mostly because the dreadful narcissist cannot see himself reflected back from her 'so totally different were her delicate features and mild dark

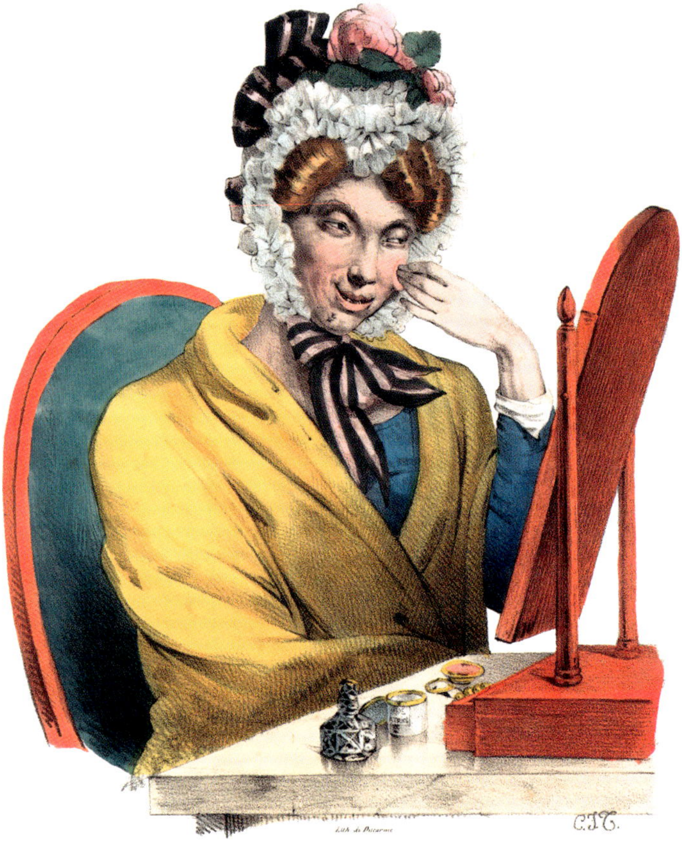

'Who will be able to resist me?', French satire *c.* 1820. Many products made extravagant anti-aging claims, which many hopeful people spent a fortune on in their desire to retain a youthful appearance.

eyes from his own'. Even so, 'a few years before Anne Elliot had been a very pretty girl, but her bloom had vanished early' so now that she was 'faded and thin there was nothing to excite his esteem'. His judgement of his favourite daughter, Elizabeth, was slightly less harsh as fortunately 'she is still the same handsome Miss Elliot that she had begun to be thirteen years ago'. Nevertheless, Elizabeth is becoming concerned for her future: 'She had the consciousness of being nine-and-twenty ... she felt her approach to the years of danger, and would have rejoiced to be certain of being properly solicited by baronet-blood within the next twelve-month or two'.

Sir Walter 'considered the blessing of beauty as inferior only to the blessing of a baronetcy'. His obsession with looks causes him to judge and criticise all around him. He judges Anne as haggard, Mary as coarse and 'the rapid increase of the crow's foot about Lady Russell's temples had long been a distress to him'. He observes that he and Elizabeth are 'as blooming as ever, amidst the wreck of the good looks of everybody else; for he could plainly see how old all the rest of his family and acquaintance were growing'. This is because he and Elizabeth share a secret: they use Gowland's lotion. Perhaps the best known of the commercially manufactured beauty products of the eighteenth century, Gowland's was an expensive cleansing lotion with a special added ingredient to its secret recipe: a dash of mercuric chloride.

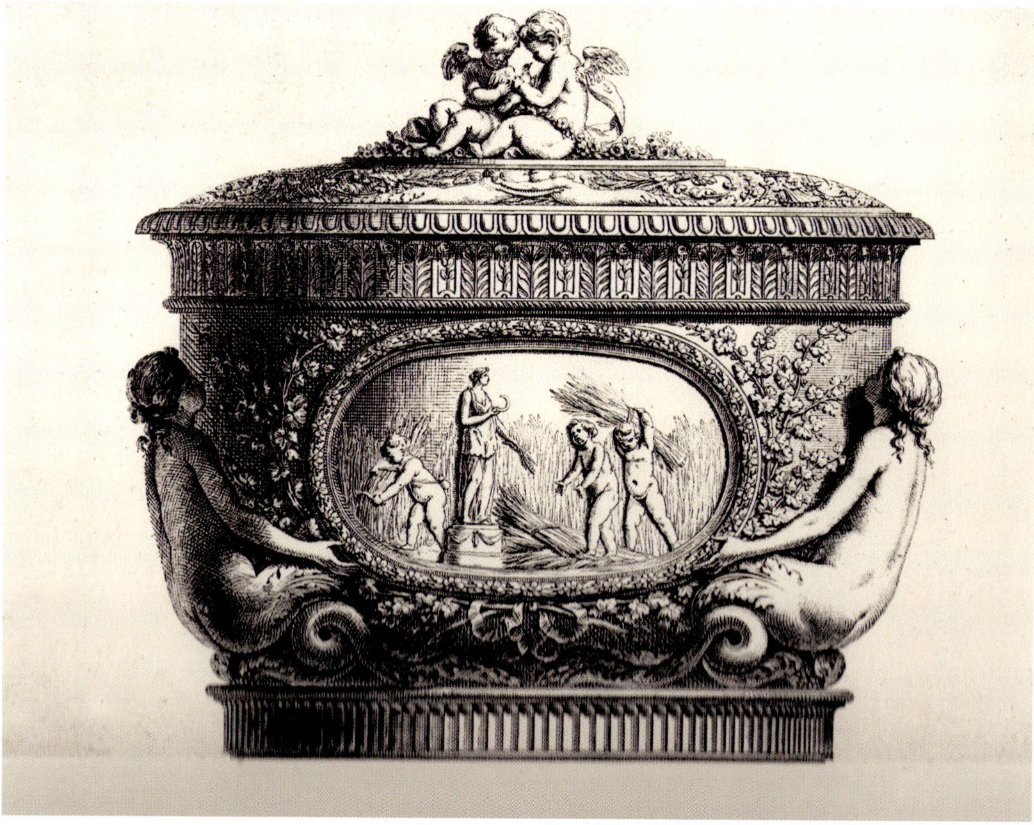

Above and right: A design for an ornamental powder box for the dressing table by Jean-François Forty as part of a series from *c.* 1764 to 1790.

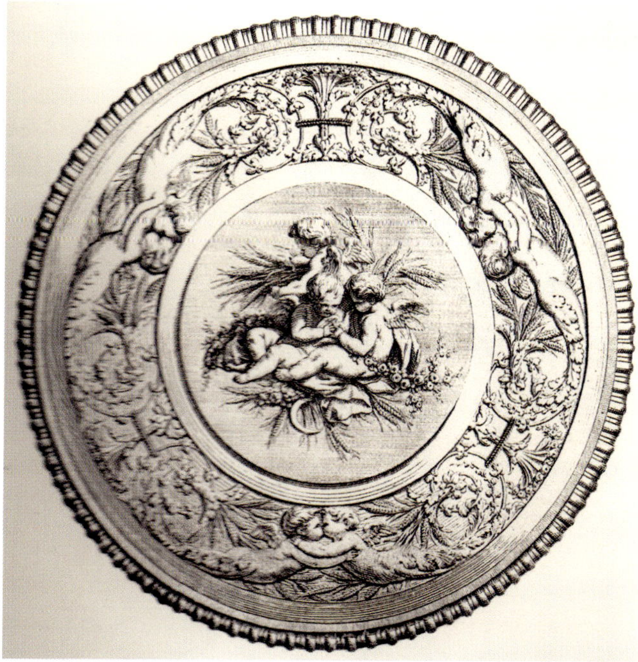

With its aristocratic clientele, Gowland's lotion had been regarded as a top-tier beauty product since the 1790s, when a number of essays extoling its virtues were published – mostly by its manufacturer, John Gowland. However, by the time Jane was writing *Persuasion* the claims and the product had largely been discredited. In 1807, Robert Thomas MD revised his *The Modern Practice of Physic*, including the note: 'A remedy much employed by women who are troubled with eruptions in the face is Gowland's lotion, the basis of which is generally supposed to be muriated quicksilver; but it is a hazardous application when continued for any length of time.'

It is with this irony that she underlines the foolish vanity of Sir Walter who ignores Anne until an unexpected improvement in her dowdy looks piques his interest. He considers that she suddenly seems 'less thin in her person, in her cheeks; her skin, her complexion, greatly improved; clearer, fresher' and perhaps even 'the bloom and freshness of youth restored'. He wonders 'Had she been using any thing in particular?' and upon hearing no,

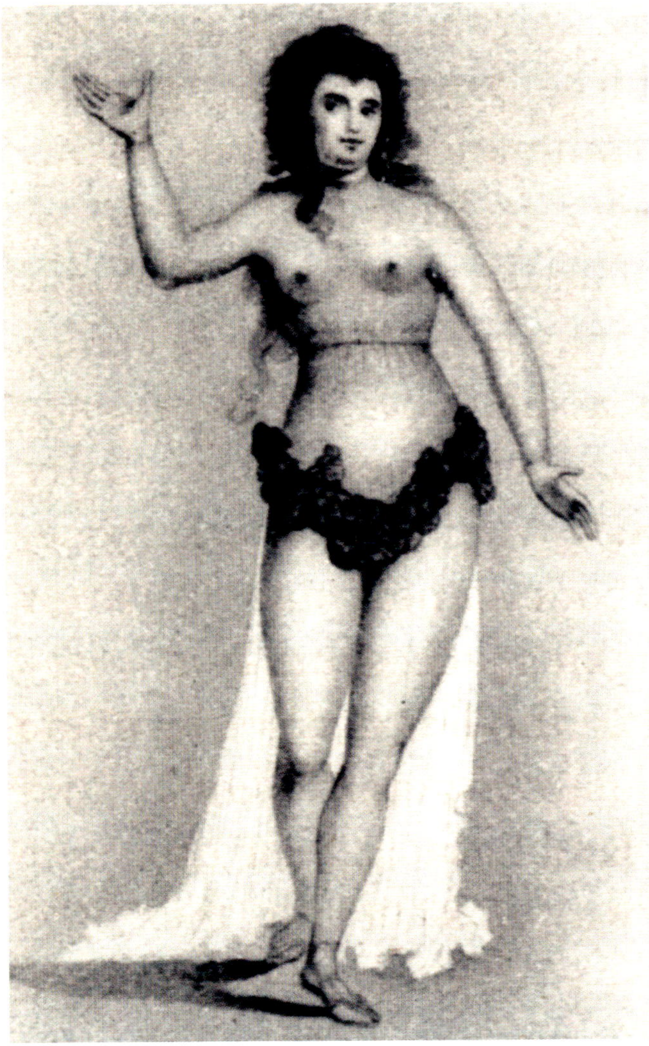

Miss Chudleigh in her scandalously sheer costume as Iphigenia, 'undressed for the sacrifice'.

nothing at all, he assures himself 'Merely Gowland'. He does not consider for one second that Anne's bloom might have been restored from within, as she begins to have hope that she might actually have love in her future.

In his essay 'Epitome of a Manuscript Essay on Cutaneous Diseases' of 1794, John Gowland revealed that he had invented his lotion for the notorious aristocratic beauty Elizabeth Chudleigh, the Duchess of Kingston, who, aged only eighteen, came to serve as lady in waiting to the Dowager Princess of Wales. Her most infamous stunt was an appearance at a masquerade in 1749 in the costume of Iphigenia 'undressed for the sacrifice', her wisp of a costume so diaphanous that it was said she appeared naked.

Unfortunately, when Gowland met her she was suffering a severe breakout, 'her skin became affected with a lumpy thickness and opacity ... she had recourse to paints, patches, and cosmetics, of every denomination' which had exacerbated the problem, and the medicines and sea-bathing prescribed by the royal physicians did nothing. Only Gowland could save her with his miraculous lotion, which of course became a toilette essential for all the court once they saw how it had restored her beauty!

As well as claiming her endorsement, he used his leaflet to explain how Gowland's lotion should be used:

> Its first object being to excite in a small and temporary degree an apparent increase of the eruption which it finally cures and eradicates ... [it] extracts the thick and turgid virus lurking in the interior fibres and brings it forward to the surface in the form of a SCURF or whitish powder which every morning falls or is wiped off until the skin by being thus frequently purified and from day to day purged of its crudities.

No doubt Elizabeth Chudleigh's rivals would have gossiped about the possibility that she might have contracted her skin problem from one of her many affairs, but it might have been damage from the corrosive quality of the white lead in ceruse, or possibly the result of the poisonous make-up improperly removed and clogging the pores of the skin. Either way, as Gowland promised, the mercuric chloride in Gowland's lotion would have stripped the outer layers of the epidermis like a chemical peel to reveal fresh new layers of skin beneath. Unfortunately, he did not reveal that with continued use it could cause increased salivation and bad breath, as well as inflammation and ulceration of the mucous membranes resulting in respiratory problems, abdominal pain, kidney failure and possibly even death.

It certainly would have answered the problem of effective make-up removal, as many women who used ceruse reported sensitivity to soap. This was hardly surprising as many soaps were extremely harsh, and it wasn't until after the cessation of the punitive Soap Tax that companies like Pears (founded in 1807) started to produce gentle vegetable-based soaps.

Renowned rival product Bloom of Ninon also made abundant claims in their advertising but unfortunately neglected to mention that, along with the essence of lavender and almond emulsion, the ingredients included white lead. 'It is particularly recommended for the hands and arms, bestowing on them a delicacy and whiteness, superior to any thing vended for similar purposes.'

There was also Sicilian Bloom of Youth and Beauty, which claimed to be 'as innocent as milk: this impalpable Powder, while it communicates to the Skin the most brilliant

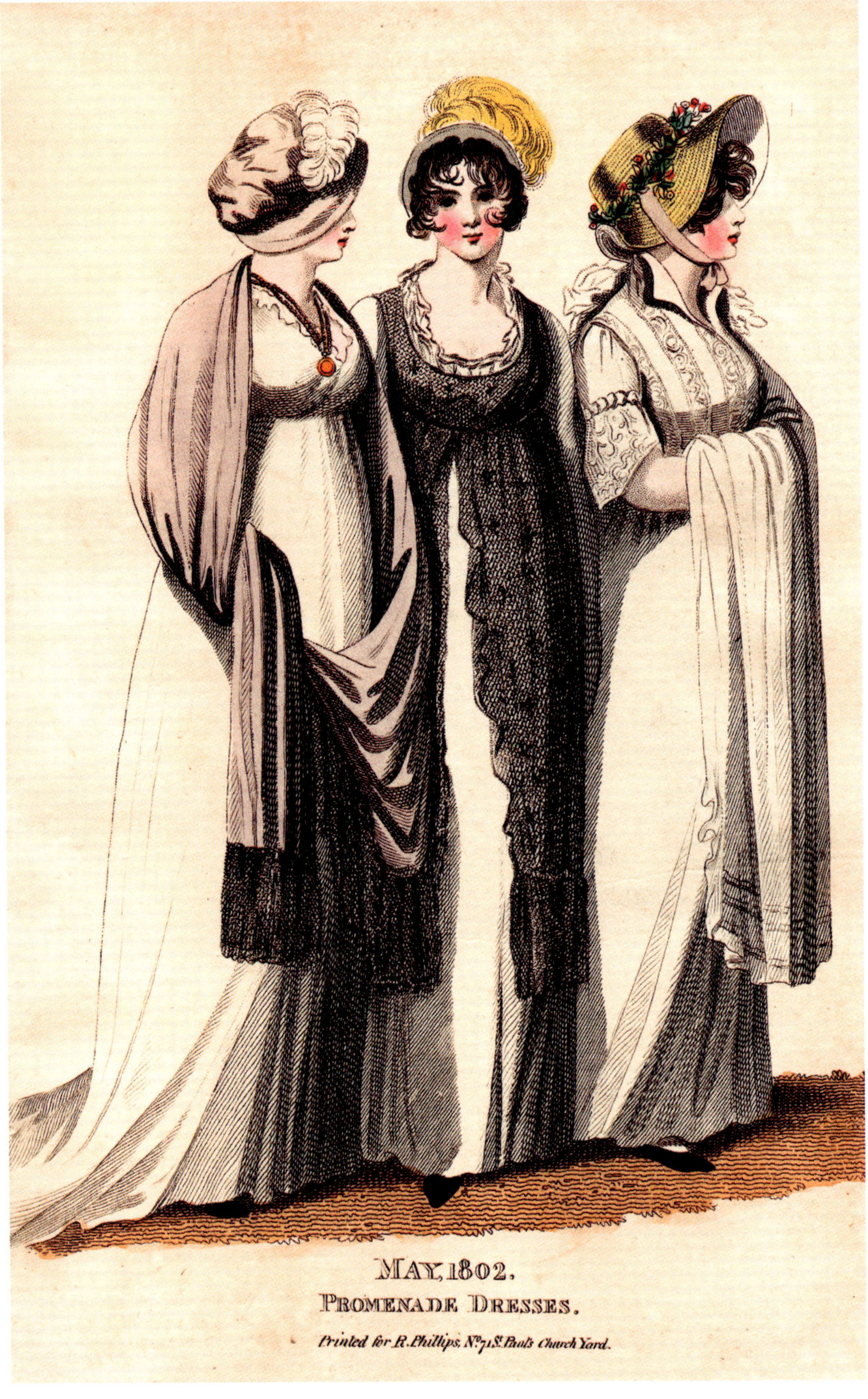

'Promenade Dresses', *The Lady's Magazine*, May 1802. There was a multitude of rouge products, mostly evoking the idea of a natural 'bloom of roses'.

Fairness, is so natural ... it cannot be detected by the most, scrutinous observer ... and so permanent, that it cannot be removed without washing'.

As well as their famous soap, Pears also launched a trio of Blooms in 1807, as advertised in *La Belle Assemblée* in October that year. Almond bloom offered a tint of natural colour, White Imperial gave a lustrous gleam and Bloom of Roses gave delicate shades of blush. Pears were also offering 'Rose colour and Pink saucers', a fascinating hybrid of cosmetic and art supply as it could be used for painting on velvet and dyeing silk as well as applied to cheek and lip!

The natural complexion might have been prized, but this was not the case for the hair or freckles it comes with! So, with the turn towards natural products, a new market for depilatories emerged. Hubert's Roseate Powder used the advertising pages of Ackermann's *Repository of Arts* in September 1809, taking a full-page ad to inform:

> 'Beautiful Women, the greatest Blemish to Female Delicacy and Beauty is Superfluous Hairs on the Face, Neck & Arms, that truly elegant and fashionable article HUBERT's Roseate Powder, IMMEDIATELY REMOVES THEM,' Hubert's state specifically that it: 'Cannot injure or inflame the SKIN, but Renders the Complexion beautifully white, delicate and fair ... Combining the splendid Advantages of an elegant Cosmetic, with the most efficacious Depilatory ever yet discovered.'

But, it has to be wondered, what was actually in a product that was applied as a cosmetic powder but that also removed hair?

Some advertisers were more willing to substantiate their claims, or at least explain them. In July 1814, Trent's Depilatory asserted that their product would remove superfluous hair in minutes and any lady who wished 'an ocular demonstration of its efficacy and innocence' could visit their premises each day between 12 and 2 p.m.

As arms were frequently on display in evening dress, depilatories were often used to remove the downy hairs to make them more like the lustrous marble of the Grecian statues so admired at the time. When removing hair from the arms, it is unlikely that the underarms would be neglected, but none of the advertisers mention anything more specific than the intriguing 'and other parts'.

Grey hair was a great fear for all, as it suggested the end of vitality and the harbinger of decrepitude. A number of hair dyes began to appear, each promising to be safe and harmless – not like earlier dyes that used corrosive substances like lye. It was also used to get rid of red hair, which, due to the unfavourable association with Judas Iscariot, was considered almost as bad as grey.

Famous for their Bear's Grease pomatum, Atkinson's also offered a vegetable dye 'for changing Red or Grey hair to an Auburn or Black', as did De Veau's indelible fluid, which promised to transform hair, eyebrows and whiskers from the embarrassing shades of grey or red to beautiful shades of flaxen brown or black, boasting that 'the eyebrows and whiskers are changed in two hours – the application is so easy that any lady may accomplish it herself; yet so exquisite is the change that the most penetrating eye cannot discover it to be the effect of art'.

One of the most terrifying blights to beauty was a lost tooth – nothing declared age and decrepitude more resolutely. There were, however, a wide variety of artificial teeth

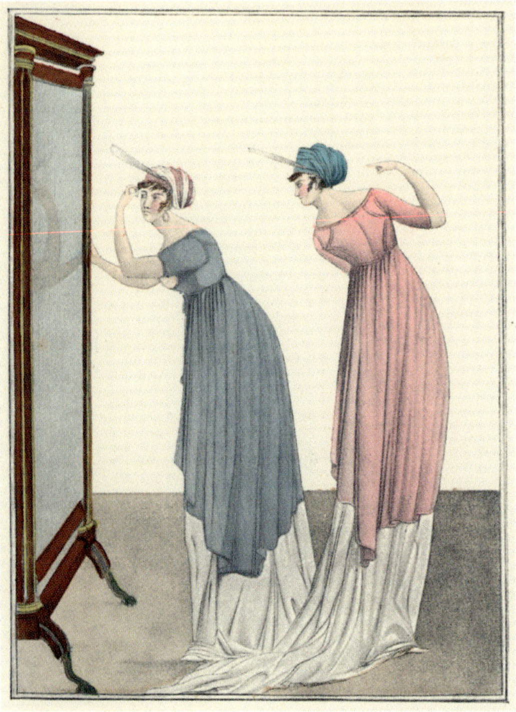

Left: 'Evening Dresses from Hamburger Moden und Elegance', 1802. They are wearing elegant Mamalouc caps but their arms are bare so they might be in need of a depilatory!

Below: *A Wig Shop* (Thomas Rowlandson, *c.* 1790). Two mature ladies are being flattered into trying wigs of pretty youthful styles, no doubt in the hope that they will help them look younger.

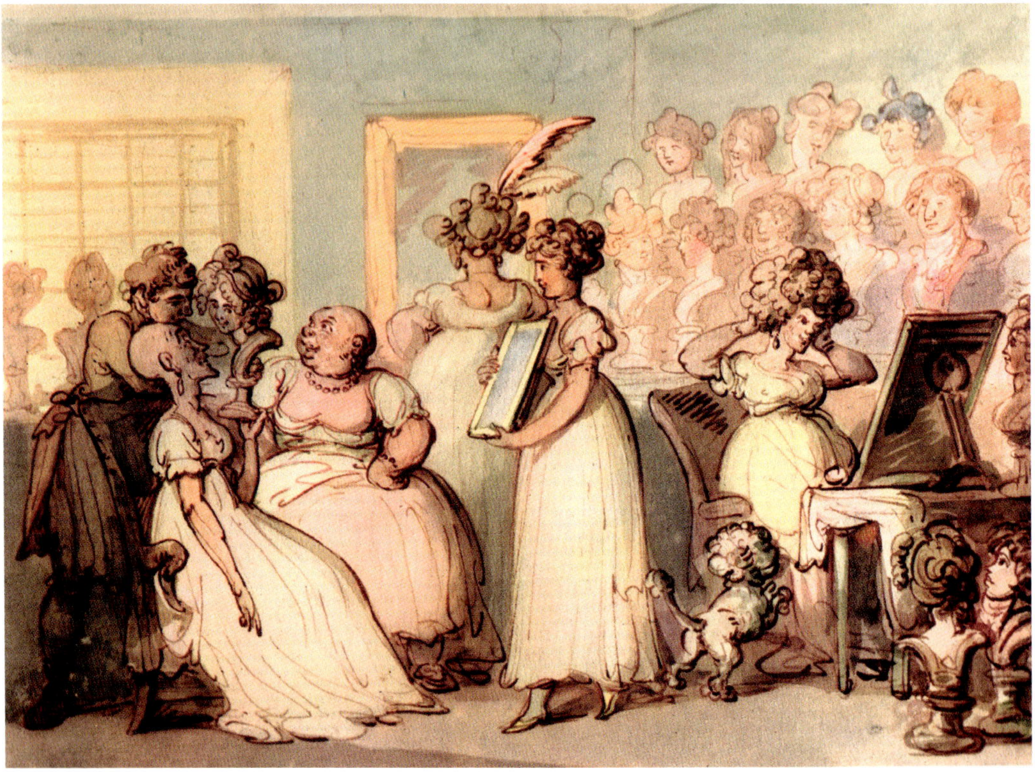

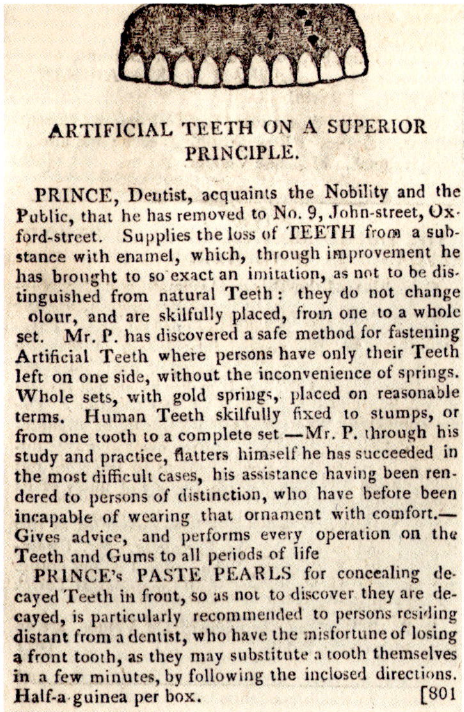

ARTIFICIAL TEETH ON A SUPERIOR PRINCIPLE.

PRINCE, Dentist, acquaints the Nobility and the Public, that he has removed to No. 9, John-street, Oxford-street. Supplies the loss of TEETH from a substance with enamel, which, through improvement he has brought to so exact an imitation, as not to be distinguished from natural Teeth: they do not change olour, and are skilfully placed, from one to a whole set. Mr. P. has discovered a safe method for fastening Artificial Teeth where persons have only their Teeth left on one side, without the inconvenience of springs. Whole sets, with gold springs, placed on reasonable terms. Human Teeth skilfully fixed to stumps, or from one tooth to a complete set —Mr. P. through his study and practice, flatters himself he has succeeded in the most difficult cases, his assistance having been rendered to persons of distinction, who have before been incapable of wearing that ornament with comfort.—Gives advice, and performs every operation on the Teeth and Gums to all periods of life

PRINCE's PASTE PEARLS for concealing decayed Teeth in front, so as not to discover they are decayed, is particularly recommended to persons residing distant from a dentist, who have the misfortune of losing a front tooth, as they may substitute a tooth themselves in a few minutes, by following the inclosed directions. Half-a-guinea per box. [801

Right: An advertisement for artificial teeth from the pages of *La Belle Assemblée,* November 1807.

Below: 'A French Dentist Shewing a Specimen of his Artificial Teeth and False Palettes' (Thomas Rowlandson, 1802). Artificial mineral teeth would not decay, but with lurid red gums they were obviously artificial!

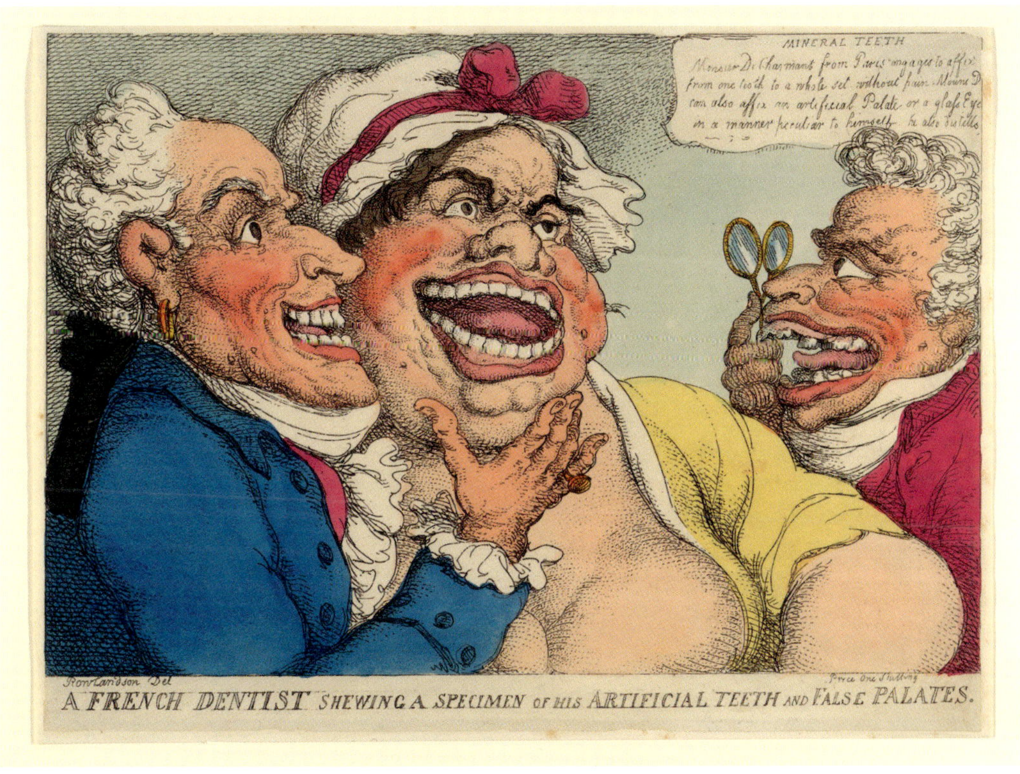
MINERAL TEETH
Monsieur De Chasmant from Paris engages to affix from one tooth to a whole set without pain. Mons. D can also affix an artificial Palate or a glass Eye in a manner peculiar to himself he also distills
Rowlandson Del
Price One Shilling
A FRENCH DENTIST SHEWING A SPECIMEN OF HIS ARTIFICIAL TEETH AND FALSE PALATES.

available by mail order. Hopeful purchasers would mould soft wax into horseshoe shapes to take impressions of the remaining teeth and the gaps between so a plate or bridge could be made to fit. Sadly, it was far from perfect, and many people suffered miserably with the discomfort of ill-fitting, artificial teeth.

Carved from hippopotamus or walrus ivory, lines of representative teeth were secured between the precious remaining teeth. Unfortunately, the ivory was subject to the same problems of decay as human teeth and even with the best care would not last much longer than a year before becoming blackened and decayed, causing accompanying foul, malodourous breath. Invented in 1788, porcelain 'mineral teeth' would not decay but unfortunately made a terrible grating noise when attempting to chew.

In 'Catharine, or The Bower' from Jane's *Juvenilia*, written in 1792 when she was seventeen, Kitty is prevented from attending a ball by a sudden vicious toothache. Her friend, Camilla, exclaims:

> Poor thing! what pain you are in! I declare it is quite Shocking to look at you. But you wo'nt have it out, will you? For Heaven's sake do'nt; for there is nothing I dread so much. I declare I had rather undergo the greatest Tortures in the World than have a tooth drawn.

Sadly, it was an experience that Jane's nieces, the daughters of Edward Austen Knight, would have in real life some years later, which Anne wrote to Cassandra about from Henrietta Street, Covent Garden, on 15–16 September 1813:

> Going to Mr Spence's was a sad Business & cost us many tears ... The poor Girls & their Teeth! ... Marianne had two taken out after all ... When her doom was fixed, Fanny, Lizzy & I walked into the next room, where we heard each of the two sharp hasty Screams ... I would not have had him look at mine for a shilling a tooth & double it. It was a disagreeable hour.

Whilst artificial teeth could help the shape of the face and clarify the speech, nothing could make artificial front teeth look convincing. There really was nothing like real, human teeth – and there were plenty available if you knew where to look.

In such an era of war and revolution, tragically there was no shortage of healthy people cut down in their prime. Horrifically, there were those who visited battlefields with pliers in hand to prise open the jaws of the fallen and steal their teeth. Known as 'Waterloo Teeth', they were sent by the barrel load to Paris or London for use in dentistry. If there wasn't a battlefield full of fresh young bodies to pilfer, those enterprising graverobbers, the resurrectionists who plundered fresh graves for corpses to sell to unscrupulous doctors, would also turn a hand to pulling teeth from them for a lucrative easy pay-off. Unpleasantly, as the teeth remain well preserved for a long time, even older graves were raided, and many a denture would have been supplied by an ancient, long-deceased, unwitting donor.

For those who were squeamish about wearing the teeth of the dead, science presented a new possibility at the end of the eighteenth century – transplantation. In keeping with the cult of scientific experimentation and the questionable medical practices of the time, tooth transplantation became all the rage in the 1780s and 1790s. This was where a

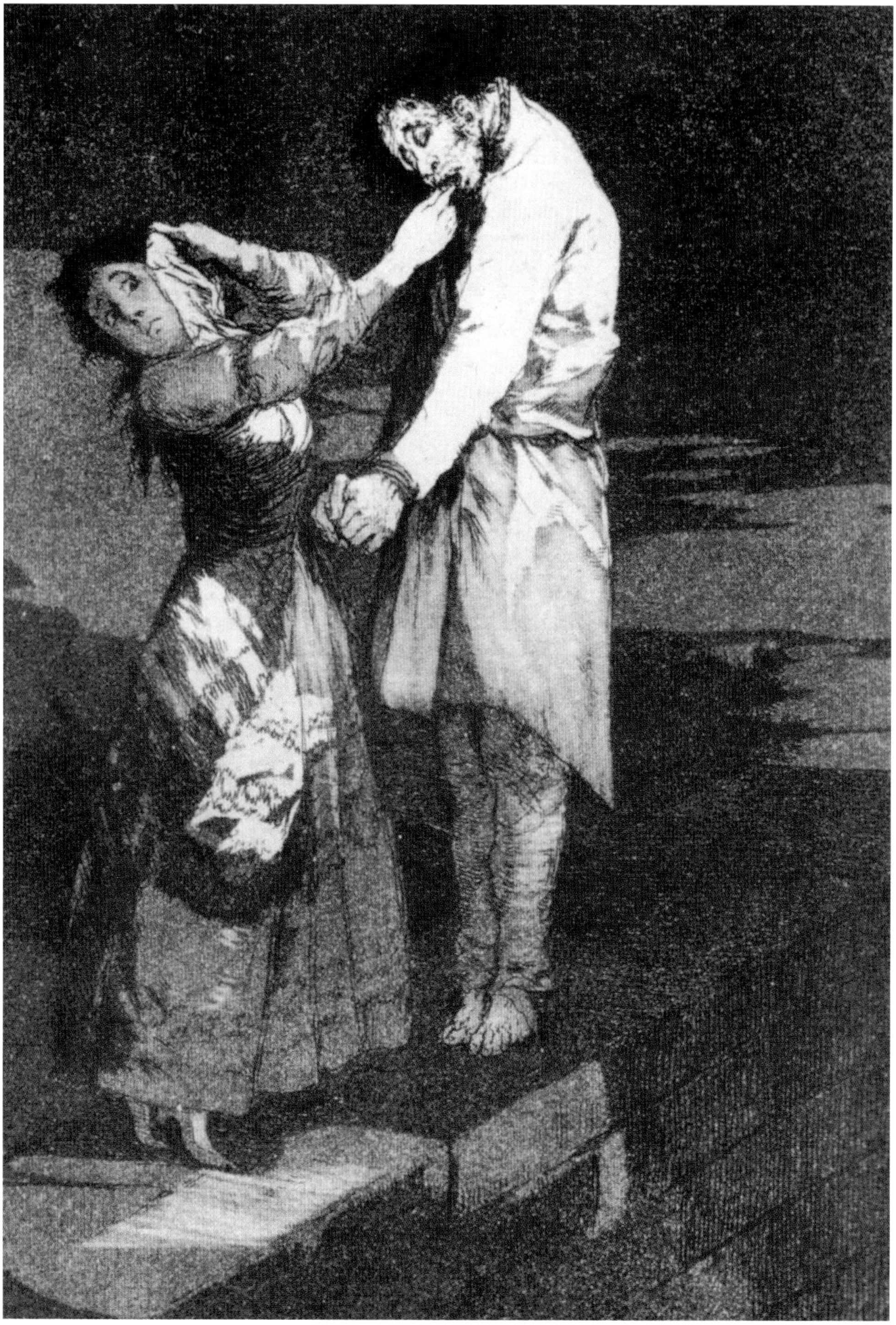

'*A Caza de Dientes*' or 'Out Hunting for Teeth' (Francisco de Goya y Lucientes, 1799). A young woman covers her face as she yanks the teeth from a hanged man. Teeth had always been valuable in witchcraft but had monetary value too in the age of tooth transplantation.

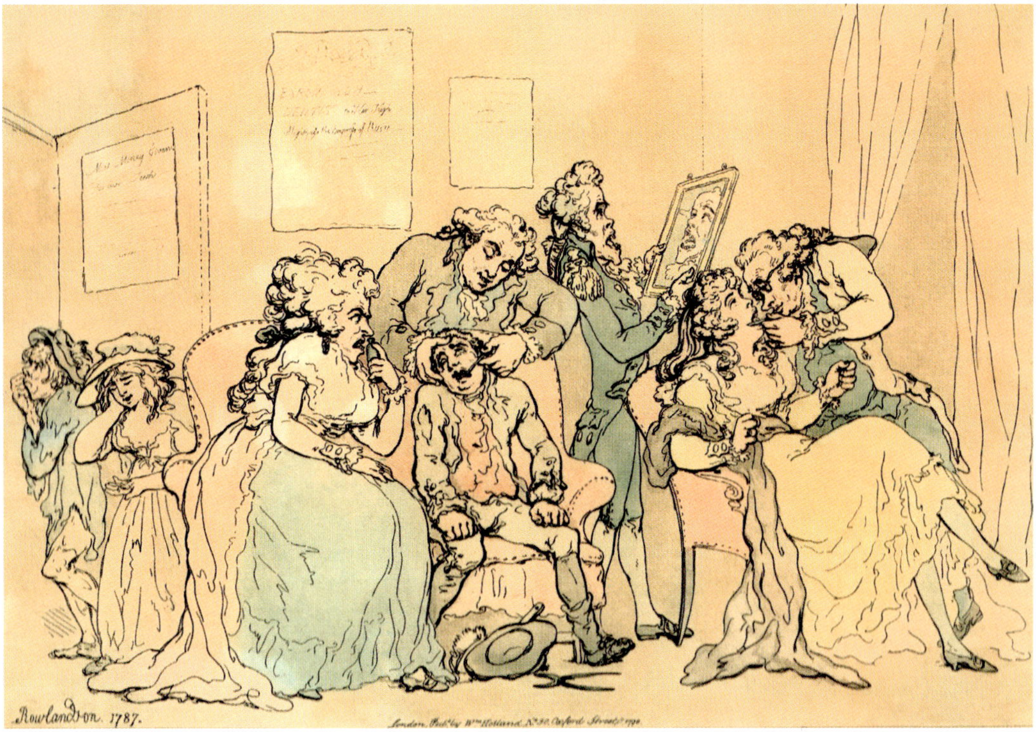

Transplanting Teeth (Thomas Rowlandson, 1787). To the left, the tragic poor leave clutching their painful empty jaws and sovereigns, whilst on the right, the wealthy are fitted with their transplants.

rotten tooth was drawn from a wealthy client whilst a healthy donor waited on hand to have the equivalent living tooth drawn fresh immediately transplanted into the waiting socket. Dentists advertised for donors and there were many attracted by the offer of up to 3 guineas for attractive front teeth. Almost all potential donors were young, healthy and, inevitably, in dire poverty.

Henry Angelo, the fencing instructor to the ton turned gossipy diarist, states in his memoir that Lady Emma Hamilton, in an early incarnation as Emma Hart, having just lost her position as servant, was in such dire straits that she was on her way to sell her teeth when he first met her. Thankfully, she was persuaded not to, although Angelo suggests that she was forced into the ignominy of joining a bawdy house in order to afford to save them. This tragic tale, or one of countless like it, would have no doubt provided inspiration for Victor Hugo to create poor Fantine in *Les Miserables* who, desperate to pay for healthcare for her child, resorted to selling her hair, her teeth and finally herself.

Surprisingly, many transplants were successful, remaining if not firmly at least in place for up to three to five years, which only encouraged the woeful trade. It was only finally when the recipient purchasers of the teeth contracted and died from syphilis from their transplanted teeth that tooth transplantation was condemned. Even so, there were still those ready to run the risk, and the last transplant recorded in Britain was in 1919.

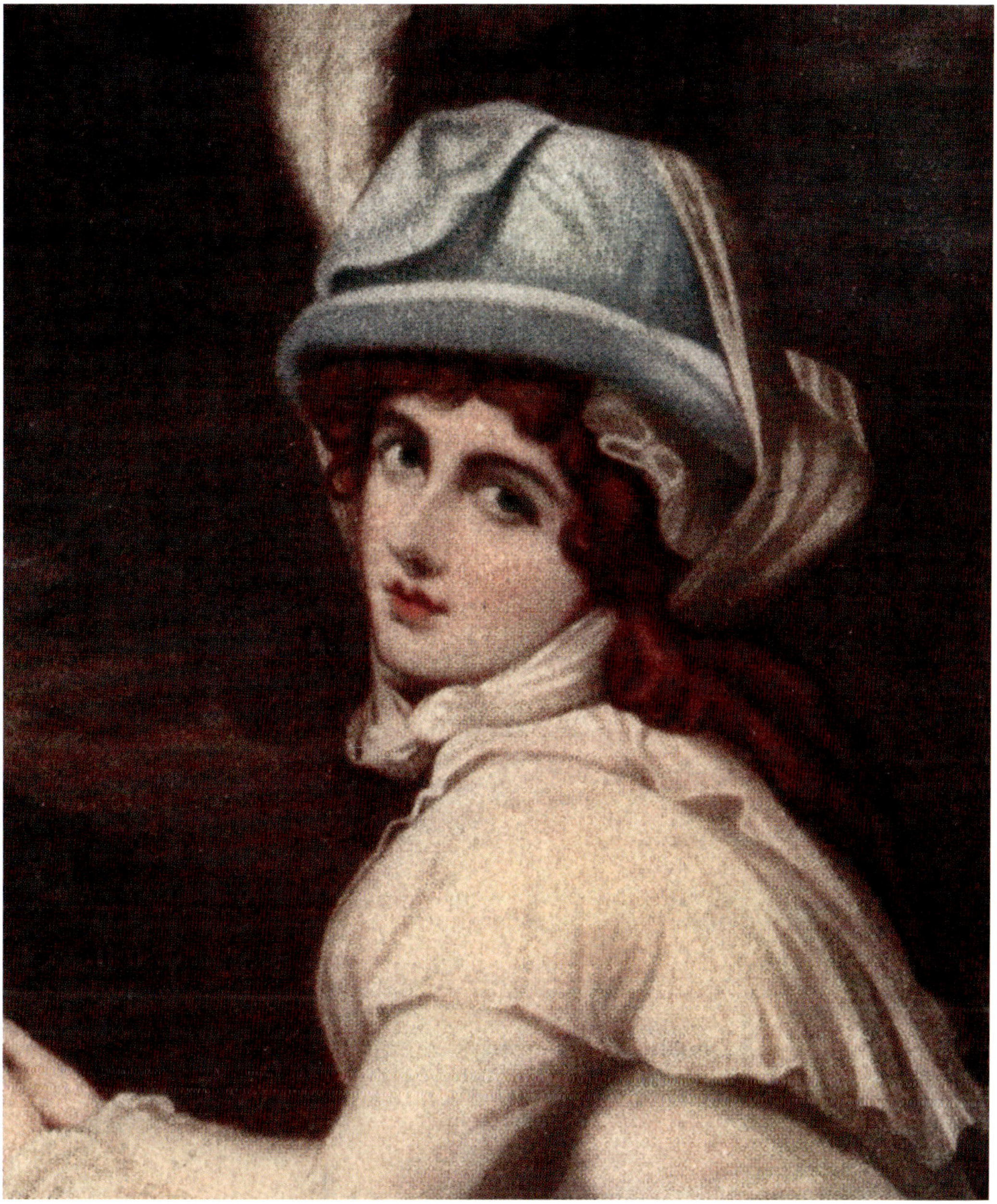

'Lady Emma Hamilton as the Ambassadress' (George Romney, 1791). The beautiful Emma was Romney's great muse, posing for him as characters from Shakespeare as well as goddesses from mythology.

4

Fresh Beauty

As Jane reflects in her novels, the most important element of beauty in the Regency era was to be like Emma Woodhouse, 'the picture of health' with a brilliant and glowing complexion. Even the plainest girl could vastly improve her looks if she would make a dedicated effort with beauty as self-improvement.

Jane frames her heroines within the range of natural beauty, and each needs to maintain her own healthy optimum to be her best, avoiding overindulgence and becoming fat, but

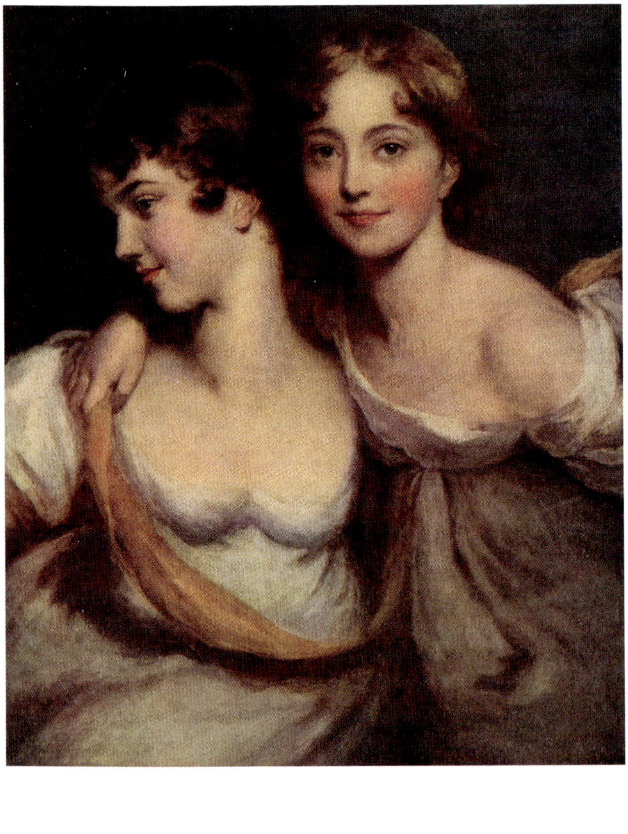

Fanny and Jane Hammond (Sir Thomas Lawrence). The sisters embody the concept of 'the picture of health'.

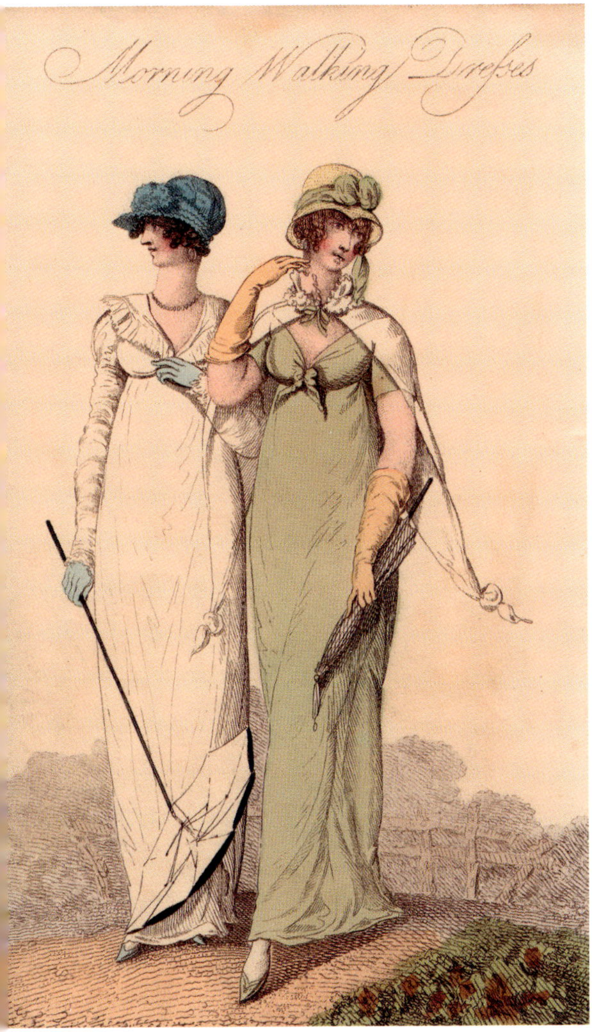

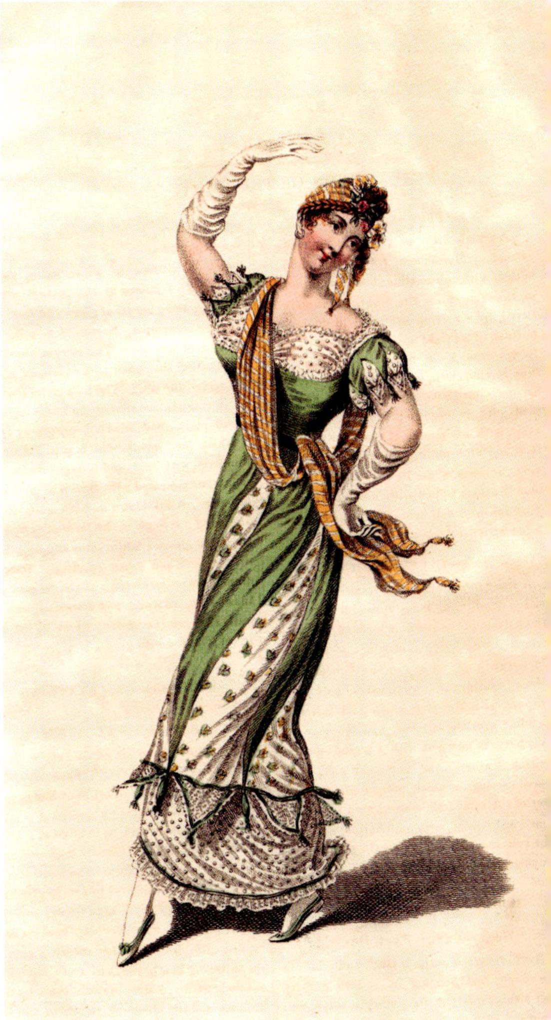

Above left: 'Morning Walking Dress', *La Belle Assemblée*, 1806. Jane characterised herself as a 'desperate walker', proud of her pace and keen to meet a challenge.

Above right: 'Fancy Ball Dress', *La Belle Assemblée*, January 1812. Jane also loved to dance: 'There were twenty dances, and I danced them all, and without any fatigue. I was glad to find myself capable of dancing so much, and with so much satisfaction as I did ... I had not thought myself equal to it, but in cold weather and with few couples I fancy I could just as well dance for a week together as for half an hour.'

equally avoiding emotional distress (if ever possible) as this will most likely cause the miserable thinness that Anne Elliot suffers from at the beginning of *Persuasion.*

There is no castigation for being plump like Harriet Smith, 'short plump and fair, with a fine bloom, blue eyes, light hair, regular features and a look of great sweetness', as being plump is also healthy and pretty. It is only the unhealthy extremes beyond that risk or suggest illness: if too thin, the risk is of consumptive diseases and looking prematurely

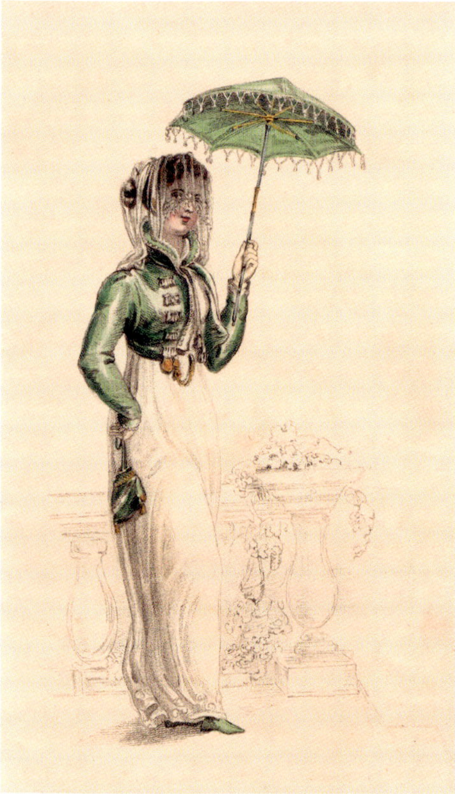 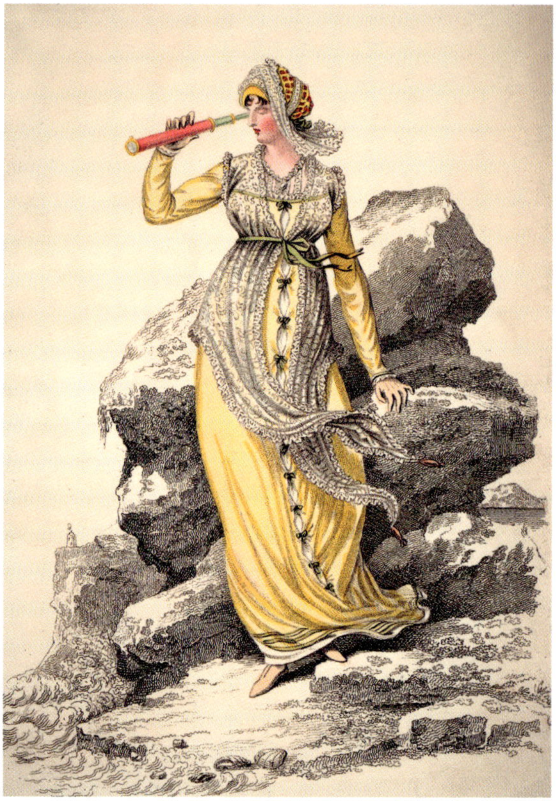

Above left: 'Promenade Dress', Ackermann's *Repository of Arts*, July 1811. She has a Chinese parasol and white veil to protect from the sun (her dress is a slightly shorter length to avoid getting muddy) and half boots – more substantial for long walks.

Above right: 'A Sea Coast Promenade Fashion', *La Belle Assemblée*, October 1809. The sea air was always regarded as 'health giving' and put natural roses in the cheeks.

old; and if plumpness exceeds *embonpoint* and runs into fat, the risk is of coronary inflammations and gout.

Throughout Jane's life the predominantly agrarian economy was strained by the Enclosures Acts, the birth of Industrialisation and the privations of war, all of which left significant portions of the population to go hungry. Therefore visible bones suggested undernourishment and all the health problems that came with it, rather than the elegance of high fashion. To have a good figure was to be the healthy ideal of your own body type rather than seeking to conform to a standard set by fashion. Ideals were set by art rather than by the example of individuals, although there was a pantheon of famous and notorious beauties who were greatly admired for their legendary beauty.

In *Pride and Prejudice* Darcy is initially indifferent to Eliza Bennet's beauty, it is only when he sees her full of health and vitality that his interest is piqued with 'admiration of the brilliancy which exercise had given to her complexion'. The rest of the household were not so enamoured: 'She has nothing, in short, to recommend her, but being an excellent walker. She really looked almost wild. ... Why must she be scampering about the country ... her hair so untidy, so blowzy and her petticoat six inches deep in mud'.

Jane was rather ahead of her time in illustrating Lizzie's health and joy coming from exercise having just walked 3 miles before breakfast. In 1825 the authors of *The Art of Beauty; or The Best Methods of Improving and Preserving the Shape, Carriage and Complexion* defined their 'Plan for Beauty-Training And Its Rules' and thereby gave hope to every girl who ever worried that she was too plain.

The authors claimed that their Plan for Beauty-Training is 'the only certain and infallible means for improving the brightness of the eyes, and the clearness and transparency of the

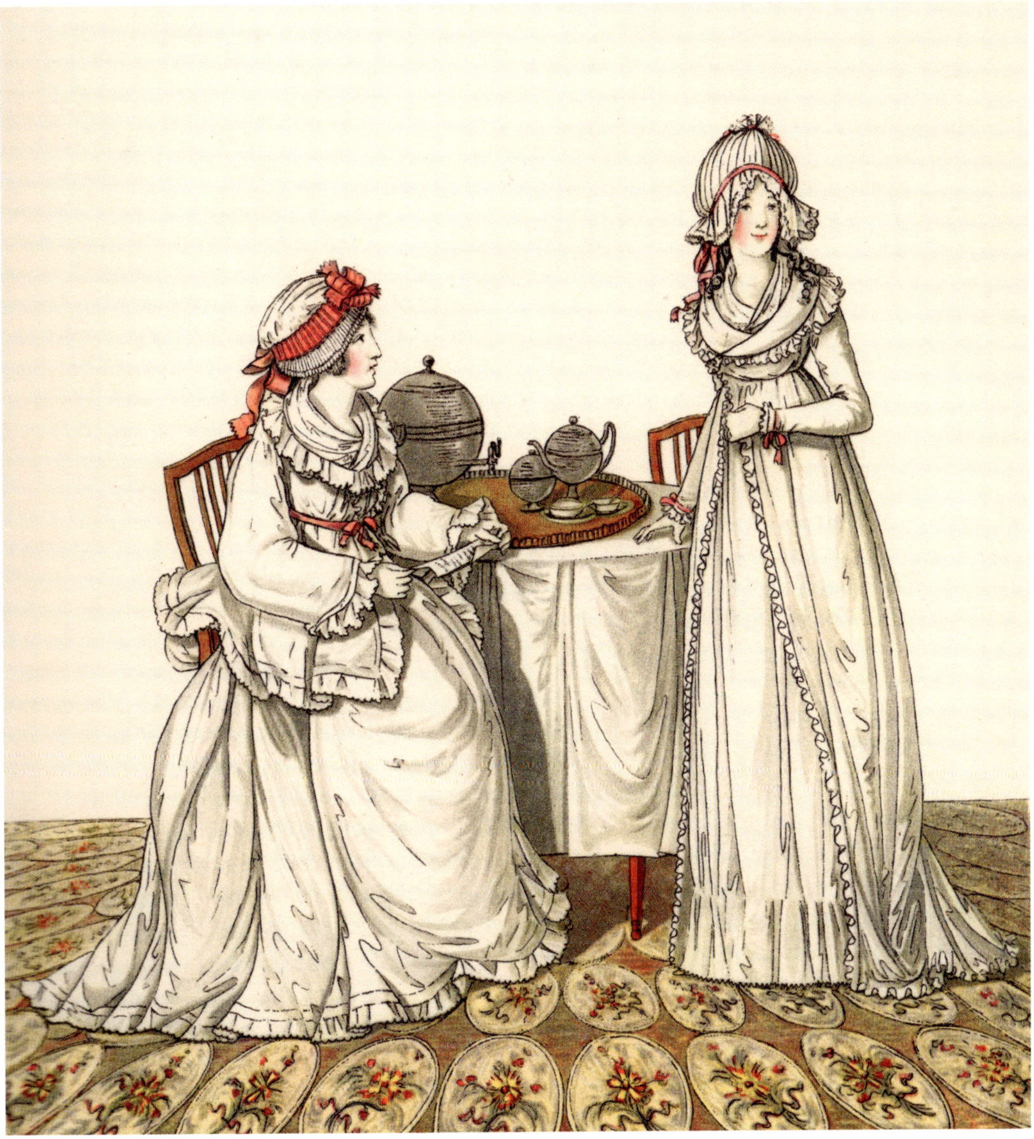

Heideloff's 'Gallery of Fashion', *c.* 1795. A fashionable breakfast was well-earned after a 3-mile walk!

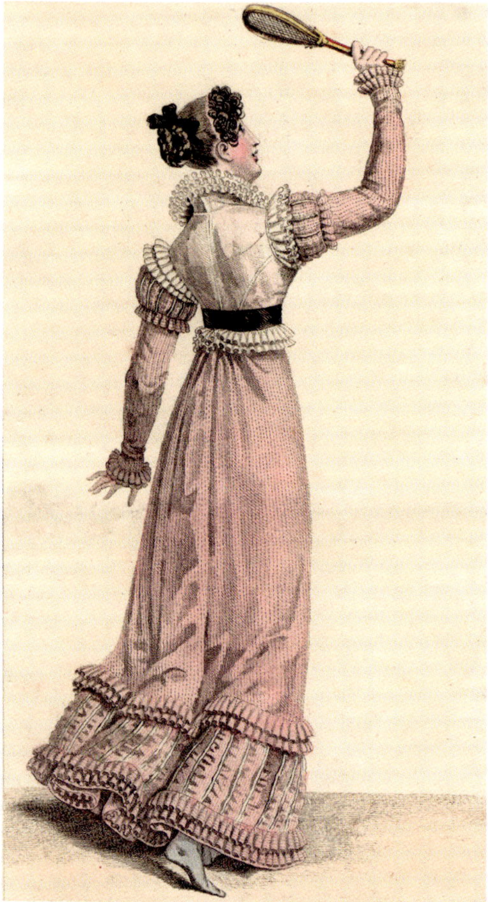

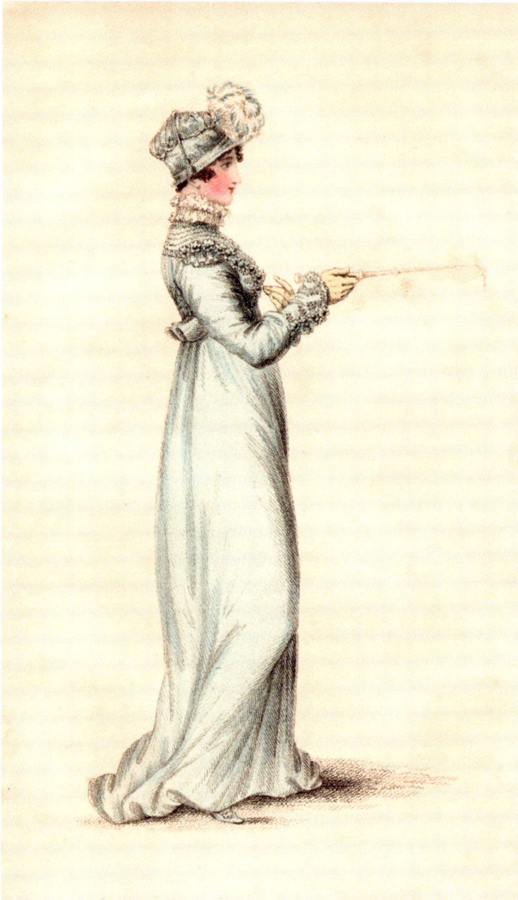

Above left: 'Costumes Parisiens', 1820. A very fashionable game of shuttlecock would be an excellent addition to the programme of exercise.

Above right: 'Ladies Riding Habit', *La Belle Assemblée*, October 1815. Riding was a popular exercise, and riding habits were usually very well cut to flatter the figure without impeding movement. Mrs Bell's design includes 'a strikingly tasteful hat which adds an air of smartness, without taking from the delicacy of a handsome face'.

complexion'. What is more, Beauty Training is the panacea that will 'remove all unhealthy, greasy, and pale-livered corpulence, and will render plump and pretty, the most meagre skeleton figure that ever was the victim of fretting, or nervous low spirits ...'.

No doubt Beauty Training could improve the complexion and the figure and bring mental health benefits but perhaps the promise of 'an additional ten years of youth, and even of restoring at least five or ten years of vanished charms' was a little extravagant!

The plan had to be rigidly adhered to for at least two months and before commencing the body must be purged with emetics and laxatives to clear the stomach and bowels, likewise the skin must be purged of all 'quack nostrums' such as Gowland's lotion or Kalydor.

To commence Beauty Training you must:

- Rise each morning at six o'clock, but not sooner.
- Before breakfast you must walk in the open air from half a mile to three miles, according to your strength, at a quick pace.
- In summer if you botanize by the way, it will be of immense advantage; or in winter, when you cannot do this, note the state of the clouds according to the classes of Mr. Luke Howard.
- If you have perspired, or if you have wetted your feet, you must change and have all dry before breakfast.
- Before breakfast it is indispensable to have your skin, well rubbed with a soft cotton cloth, or a flesh brush, for ten or fifteen minutes particularly over the stomach, and to wash your hands and face in cold soft water.
- The breakfast itself – not later than eight o'clock ought, in rigid training, to consist of plain biscuit (not bread), broiled beef steaks or mutton chops, under-done, without any fat, and half a pint of mild bottled ale, the genuine Scotch ale is the best.
- If you cannot tolerate ale, one small breakfast cup – not more – of good strong black tea or coffee – weak tea or coffee is always bad for the nerves as well as the complexion.
- If tea or coffee is taken, the half pint of ale is to be used three hours after breakfast with a biscuit, on returning from your second walk, which must be as long as the first.
- The forenoon must be spent in walking, or any other active amusement out of doors, such as gardening, nutting, romping, &c.
- Dinner at two, the same as breakfast; no vegetables, boiled meat, nor made dishes being permitted, much less fruits, sweet things, or pastry. Those who are very delicate may begin with a bit of broiled chicken or turkey, but the steaks and chops must always be the chief part of your food. A mealy potato, or a little boiled rice, may now and then be permitted, but no other vegetable.
- The afternoon should be spent in amusement in the open air, as before.
- Supper at seven or eight as most convenient, at which we allow you tea or coffee, if you have had none to breakfast; if you have, you must take your half pint of mild ale, and a bit of cold fowl, or cold roast mutton or beef, but no fat.
- Butter, cream, milk, cheese, and fish, are prohibited. You may take an egg occasionally with a biscuit.
- At meals you may eat heartily, but nothing is allowed between, not even drink.
- Thirst must be allayed without drink, by bathing the hands and face in cold water.
- You must always take at least an hour's active exercise before going to bed, and have your feet bathed in tepid water, and your whole skin rubbed with a cotton cloth or the flesh brush. Go to bed not later than ten.

Young ladies who might balk at ale for breakfast are reminded that 'this was the regular breakfast of Queen Elizabeth I and Lady Jane Grey', but after a couple of days of so much exercise, no fruit and few vegetables, they were in danger of severe dehydration and no doubt would have welcomed any liquid refreshment! The authors admit that: 'The first week or fourteen days, you may lay your account with feverishness, thirst, headache,

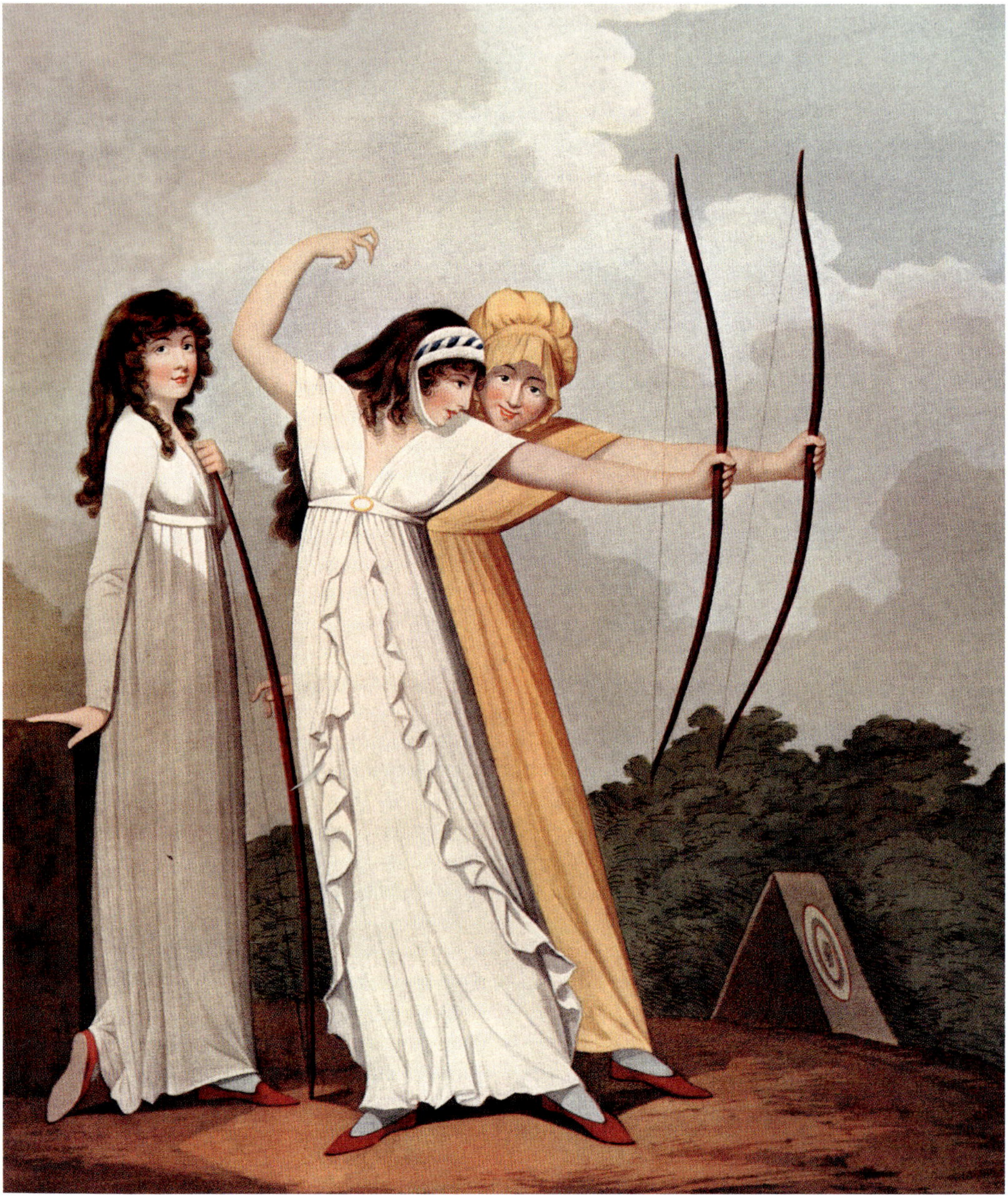

Archers (Adam Buck, 1799). Archery was to become a hugely popular sport for women during the nineteenth century.

and want of appetite; but if you persevere, this will go off, and your spirits will improve rapidly.' Clearly, they cannot imagine that their regime might be at fault as they warn: 'Recollect, that whatever rule is broken will tell to the disadvantage of the complexion, for you cannot in conscience expect improvement in beauty, while you do not pay the price of obedience.'

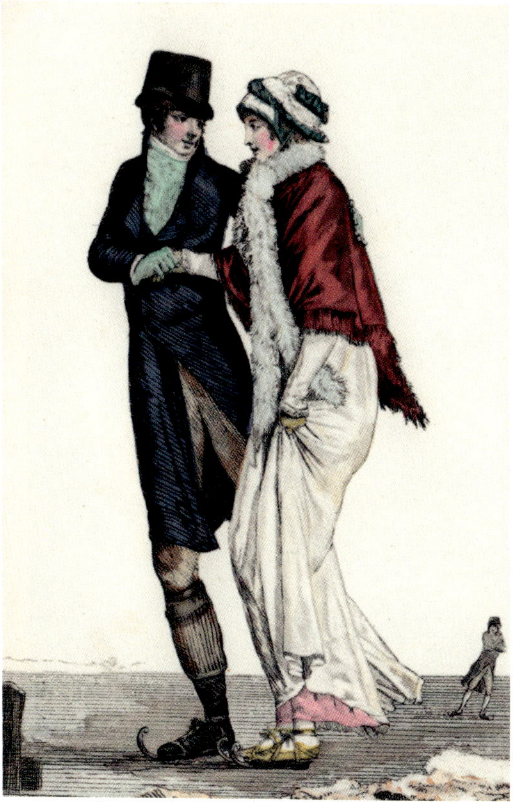

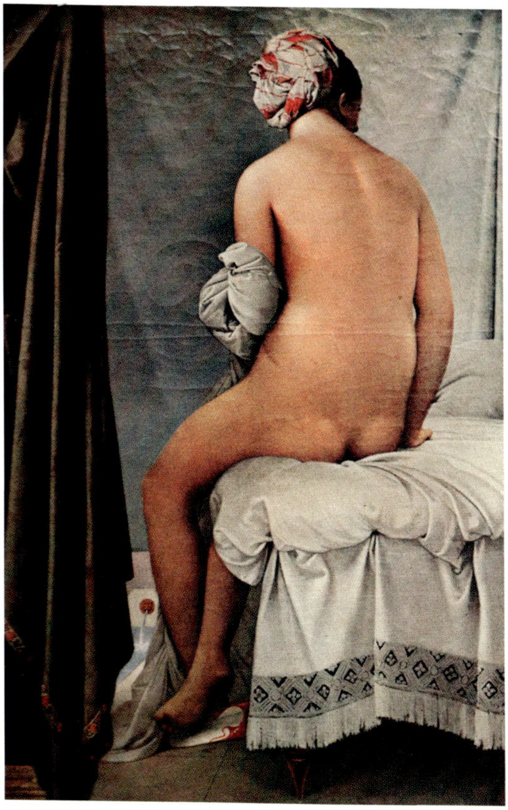

Above left: *The Timid Pupil* (Pierre De La Méssagère, *c.* 1800). At least some forms of exercise could also present the opportunity for romance!

Above right: *La Baigneuse* (Jean-Auguste-Dominique Ingres, 1808). Ingres was the first Neoclassical artist to depict nude bathers in the style of the art of Ancient Greece.

Bathing was also an essential part of Beauty Training, however it didn't have to be full immersion in water. Wealthier households had an abundance of servants to heat water and bring it to a tub by the fire, but for most people washing with a jug and basin of hot water and a sponge each day would have to suffice. Fortunately, the key part of bathing for beauty training was exfoliating: 'the brisk exercise acts like a charm upon the most harsh, rigid, and obstructed skin, while the bathing, sponging, and friction, clear away all external impurities'. They also made the more extravagant assertion that: 'No eruptions, blotches, nor pimples, even those which have baffled all medicine and medical skill, can withstand its powerful influence, but disappear as if by magic.'

5

Beauty at Home

Women in the fashionable cities were greatly blessed to be able to access the finest hairdressers and the best shops, but for everyone else a measure of domestic ingenuity had to be applied. Most Regency women including Jane Austen had a catalogue of family recipes handed down through the generations and compiled in household books. Amongst the recipes for cakes, pickles and mead were often secreted recipes for skin tonics from soured milk, scents from flowers and herbs, and even hair dyes from walnut shells. The recipes compiled within Martha Lloyd's household book used in the Austen household from the end of the eighteenth century included recipes for hand pomatum, hand soap, coral tooth powder, cold cream and lavender water, as well as Captain Austen's recipe for Milk of Roses.

Noting in *Persuasion* Sir Walter Elliot's horror at 'Admiral Baldwin, the most deplorable-looking personage you can imagine; his face the colour of mahogany ... all lines and wrinkles', it is not surprising that a sailor should have a recipe to try to improve the complexion. Captain Austen's Milk of Roses was made with: '1/2 pint of rosewater-1/2 an oz of oil of Sweet Almonds'.

Lavender water was extremely useful as a cleansing water and skin tonic as well as a fragrance and no doubt Martha Lloyd's English Lavender Water recipe was invaluable at home as well as in Jane's novels:

> In *Northanger Abbey* lavender water is referred to as part of a flirtatious conversation when Catherine and Mr Tilney are dancing and he compares the dance to marriage, and later when Eleanor is overcome by having to tell Catherine that their visit is to be cut short, Catherine soothes her with lavender water: 'Eleanor's cheeks were pale, and her manner greatly agitated. Catherine ... rubbed her temples with lavender water, and hung over her with affectionate solicitude'.
>
> In *Sense and Sensibility* lavender water is used for calming and healing, and when Willoughby snubs Marianne at the ball Elinor uses lavender water like smelling salts to try to calm her: 'Marianne, now looking dreadfully white, and unable to stand, sunk into her chair, and Elinor, expecting every moment to see her faint, tried to screen her from the observation of others, while reviving her with lavender water.'

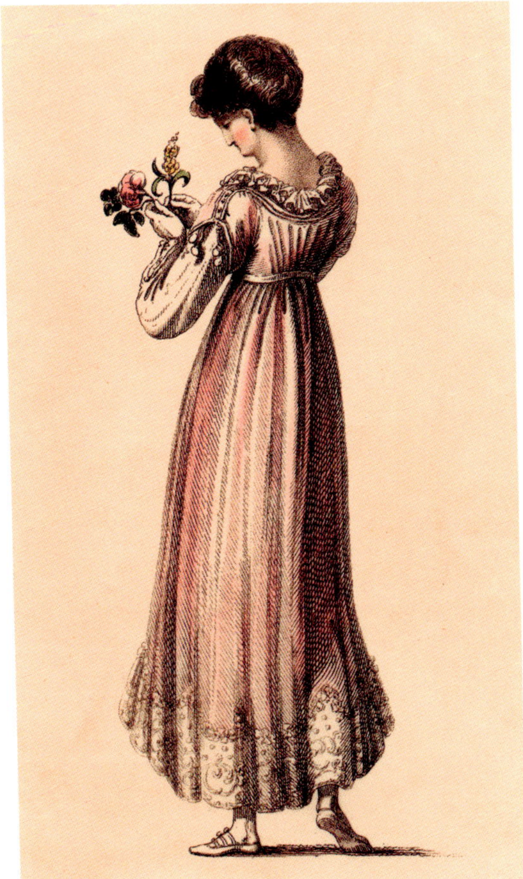

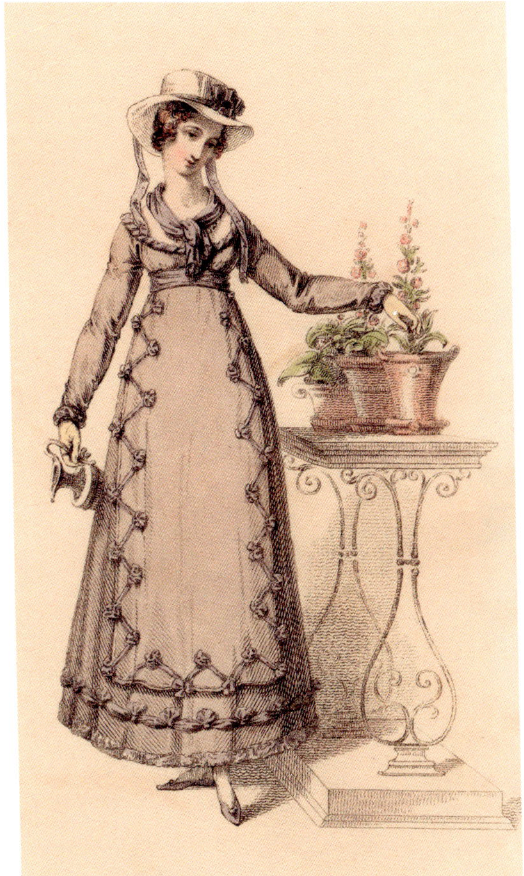

Above left: 'Evening Dress', Ackermann's *Repository of Arts,* May 1815. Beautiful pink silk frock and white triple-strapped shoes perfect for dancing, 'the hair cropped, with full curls on the forehead and in the neck'.

Above right: 'Cottage Dress', Ackermann's *Repository of Arts,* September 1820. Most women would grow a selection of herbs and flowers which would be used in all kinds of recipes.

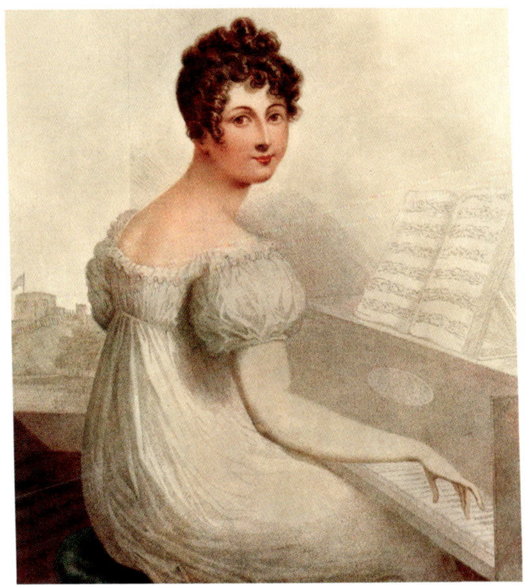

Right: The beautiful young woman playing the piano was Miss Elizabeth Conyngham, who became Marchioness Conyngham when she became the last of King George IV's lovers. She was renowned for her beauty and her avaricious nature (after J. Barrow, 1 June 1821).

Elinor relied on the calming effects of lavender again later when Marianne: 'in restless pain of mind and body ... growing more and more hysterical ... Some lavender drops, however, which she was at length persuaded to take, were of use ...'.

To augment family wisdom there had been a growing catalogue of household manuals and recipe books published since the late sixteenth century, many of them so renown that they were translated and sold widely across Europe. Written in 1772, '*The Toilet of Flora, or A Collection Of The Most Simple And Approved Methods Of Preparing Baths, Essences, Pomatums, Powders, Perfumes And Sweet Scented Waters*' was one of the most influential beauty books of the eighteenth century, running to many editions and revisions. The author, Pierre-Joseph Buc'hoz, informs that his intention is to help the Fair Sex: 'the Improvement of their Persons is the indispensable Duty of those who have been little favoured by Nature'. However, his book would still be of use to pretty women to learn the secrets of how to 'extend the Empire of their Beauty ... and ... give Force and Lustre to their Perfections'.

Over 280 recipes were included many of which are undoubtedly recipes that originated with women. These range from the charming 'A Water to change The Eyebrows Black' to

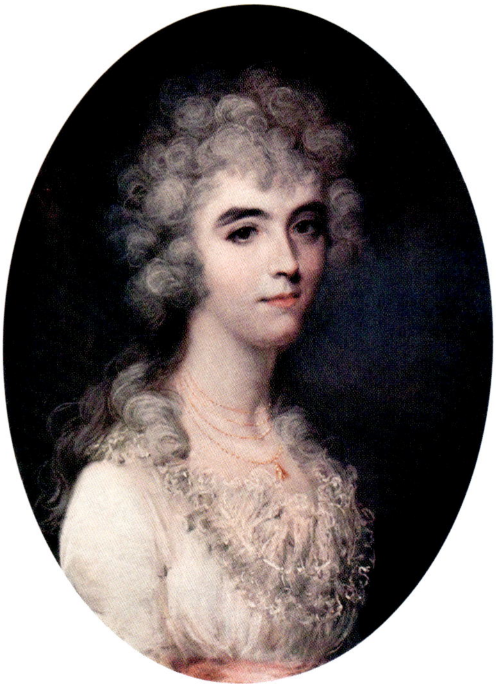

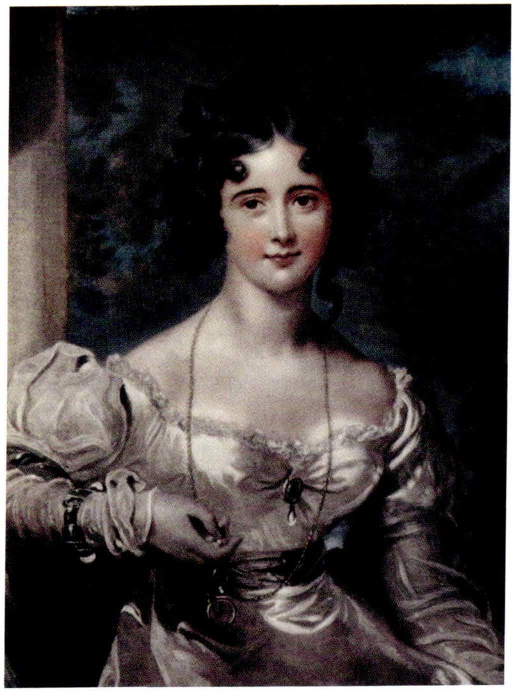

Above left: Mrs Best, daughter of General Woods Russell (John Russell RA). Her eyebrows were likely darkened with charred cloves as cloves were readily available, and the results were successful enough to last all evening.

Above right: Miss Rosamond Croker (Sir Thomas Lawrence, 1827). When this portrait was exhibited at the RA 'men stood before it in a half-circle admiring its loveliness'. This was the perfect response as the portrait was to herald Rosamond's presentation at court, announcing her launch on the marriage market.

the terrifying 'An Excellent Preservative Balsam against the Plague' and that is before the appendix of a further forty recipes for household stain removers and snuff!

There are a wide variety of cosmetic waters including the essential: 'A Cosmetic Water, of great Use to prevent Pits after the Small-Pox', and 'A Simple Balsamic Water, which removes Wrinkles', it preserves the bloom of youth, and if used only once a day, it takes away wrinkles, and gives the skin a surprising lustre.

Anyone put off by the acidic Green Vitriol in the Water to change the Eyebrows black' might try rubbing them with charred cloves or Frankincense as: 'This Black will not melt nor come off by sweating'. You could also try the recipe including melon seeds and water lilies that would 'Remove Worms in the Face' and the 'Admirable Varnish for the Skin', a concoction including lemon juice and egg whites that should be applied after washing the face with distilled water of rice, this would 'render the complexion fair, and the skin smooth, soft, and shining'.

The *Mirror of the Graces* followed in 1811, written by 'A Lady of Distinction' whose stance was firmly anti-cosmetics, with one slight exception: 'A little vegetable rouge tinging the

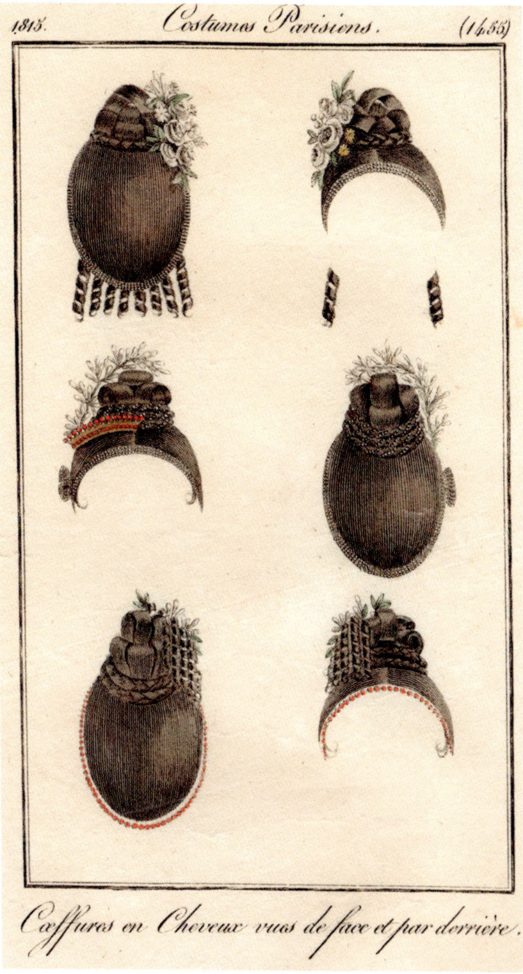
1815.
Costumes Parisiens.
(1455)
Coiffures en Cheveux vues de face et par derrière.

Coiffures from 'Costumes Parisiens', 1815. There was such interest in having the latest hairstyles that 'Costumes Parisiens' included the occasional coiffure plate.

cheek of a delicate woman, who, from ill-health or an anxious mind, loses her roses, may be excusable... like a cheerful smile on the face of an invalid, put on to give comfort to an anxious friend'. She recommends a little harmless carmine delicately applied to the areas where a blush would occur if the cheek was healthy, and definitely not in the French style, daubed on from jawline to eyelash. The strong shades of carmine red could be softened with the addition of white hair powder or a more delicate version of the colour could be extracted from fabric dyed with kermes.

So much of beauty was creating a flattering and fashionable hairstyle. Bear's Grease and Macassar oil would nourish and condition the hair, and if you believed the advertisements, would also ensure luxurious growth and that it would never break off or go grey! But what if you had lank hair like Catherine Morland in *Northanger Abbey*, or limp oily hair like many experiencing the vicissitudes of teenage hormones?

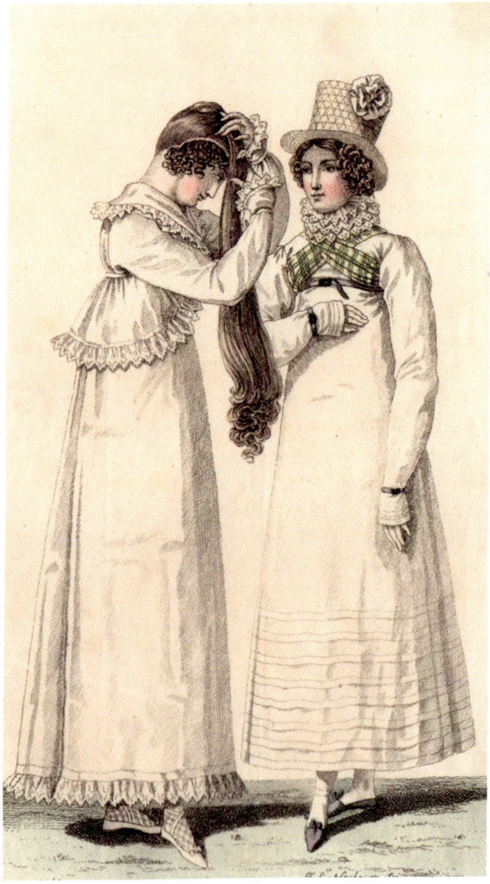

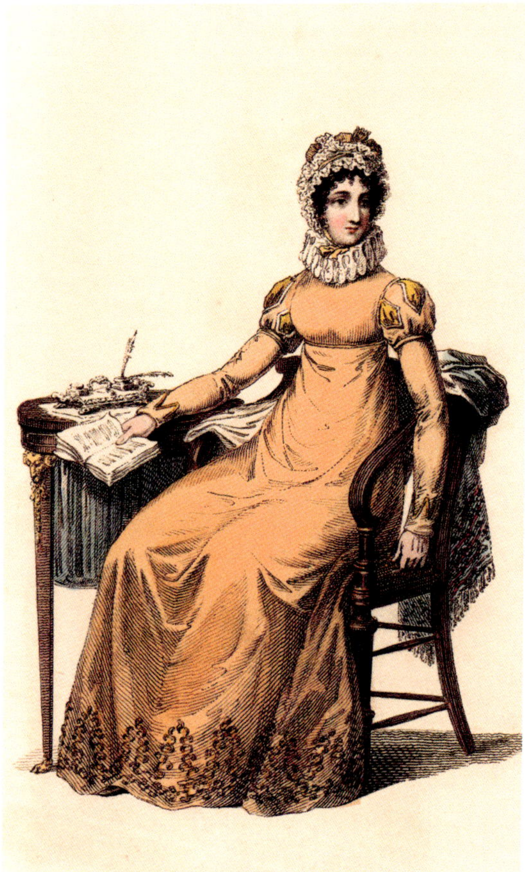

Above left: To minimise the 'torment as to hairdressing' many women, like Jane, maintained long hair with only a section at the front kept short and curled prettily to frame the face. This style was ideal for wearing caps and bonnets. ('Costumes Parisiens', 1815)

Above right: 'Morning Dress', Ackermann's *Repository of Arts*, May 1822. Jane's niece Caroline noted that Aunt Jane always wore a cap.

With the fashion for glossy ringlets and curls there was so much more reliance on the natural texture of hair. Those with straight, fine or unruly hair would resort to a regime of wearing curling papers to bed every night to maintain the memory of their chosen curls like Emma Woodhouse: 'the hair was curled and the maid sent away, and Emma sat down to think and be miserable'.

In her letters Jane relates she endures 'a world of torment as to hairdressing' so it is fitting that she has Emma dwelling in her misery as she submits to her curling papers. Jane was far from enamoured with her own hair, sharing in a letter to Cassandra: 'my short hair curls well enough to want no papering' while her long hair could be plaited up and concealed by a cap. This was a style that worked well for her with various evening ensembles, and clearly as detailed in many of her letters, she took considerable pleasure in creating a variety of caps to refresh her look. The fashion for chic evening caps, bandeaux and headdresses continued in a variety of classically inspired incarnations that endured throughout the 1790s and well into the next century.

Jane's niece Caroline recalled 'she always wore a cap – Such was the custom with ladies who were not quite young – at least of a morning – but I never saw her without one, to the best of my remembrance either morning or evening.' It seems that even aged only twenty-three Jane was unbothered by being thought to be frumpy, and simply unwilling to spend much time on the torment of her hair at home or in informal settings when she could be spending time more productively or enjoyably.

Not all her caps were frumpy, she mentions borrowing a Mamalouc cap, like a satin turban with a feather plume, and in November 1800 she wore a fashionable bandeau: 'Charlotte and I did my hair, which I fancy looked very indifferent, nobody abused it, however, and I retired delighted with my success'.

Fashionable hair dressing could be hugely time consuming and potentially dangerous. Even if curling papers were used, crimping irons, the predecessor of curling tongs, were usually used to set and finish the hairstyle. As Stewart wrote in *Plocacosmos,* the hot irons were applied to the hair until it smoked, when the curl was pinned and left to cool. This would have been damaging enough, but given that the irons were heated in the fire, there was no possibility of regulating how hot they actually got. Hair was frequently burned, not to mention scalps, ears and maid's hands!

Given the arduous nature of hairdressing, it is no surprise that many women were delighted to take the freedom of the crop. Jane's niece Anna cut all her hair off aged fifteen at a time when convention dictated that she should be making the most of her beauty in advance of her social debut. This was regarded as an act of defiance by many in the family and Jane wrote in a letter to Cassandra: 'Anna will not be surprised that the cutting off of her hair is very much regretted by several of the party in this house'. Perhaps having a little more empathy for a young woman wishing to make her own choices – or as the Rice Portrait would indicate, having had cropped hair herself as a girl – Jane was more forgiving, adding ' I am tolerably reconciled to it by considering that two or three years may restore it again'. Even if she did identify with Anna's need for self-expression, Jane was not enamoured of the effect and later wrote of Anna's 'sad cropped head'.

Cropped hair might have met with disapproval within the Austen family, but it was fashionable and appeared regularly in fashion magazines on both sides of the Channel from the time of the French Revolution until the 1810s. Worn both by women and men,

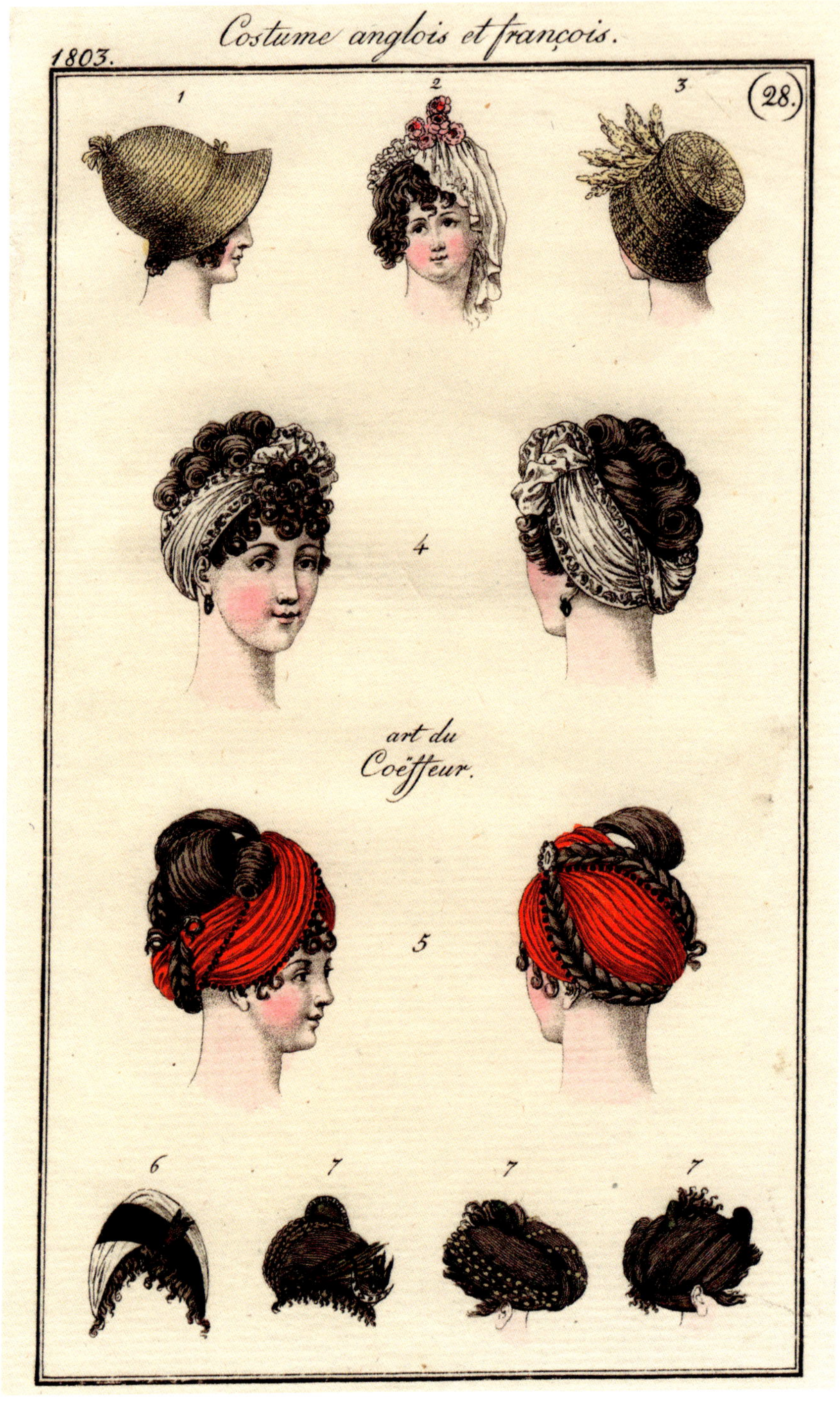

'Art de Coiffure', 'Costumes Parisiens', 1803, showing styles with artfully wrapped bandeau. Jane wore something similar at a ball in 1800: 'I wore at the ball your favourite gown, a bit of muslin of the same round my head, bordered with Mrs. Cooper's band, and one little comb.'

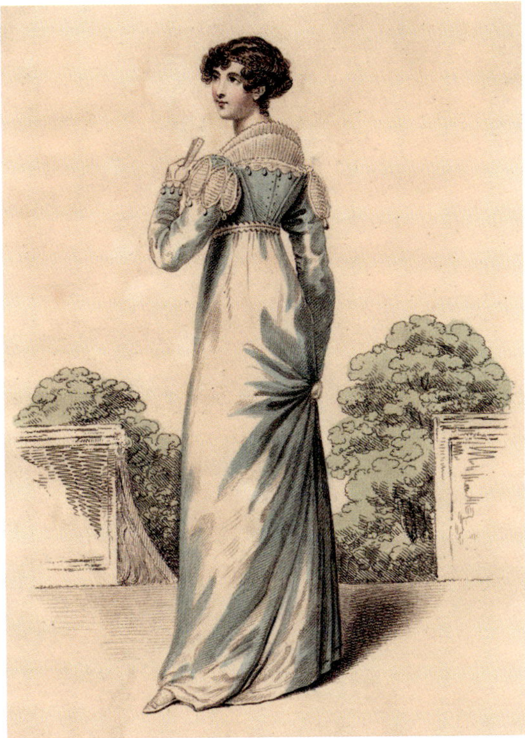

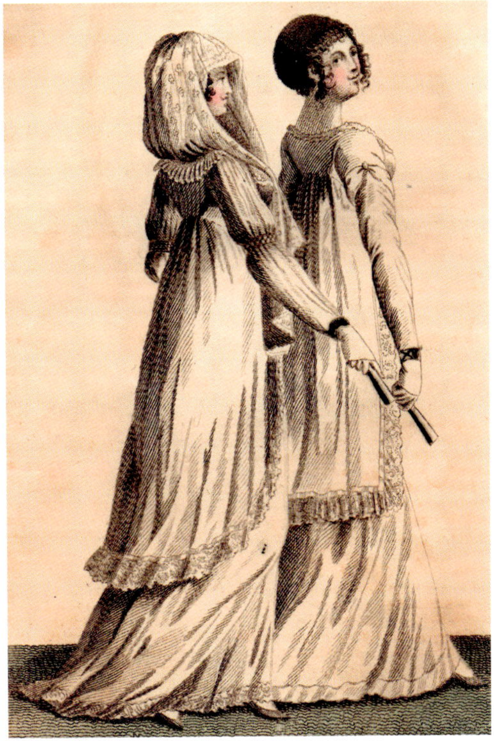

Above left: 'Half Full Dress', *La Belle Assemblée*, July 1813. Cropped curls with a plaited band around the forehead.

Above right: Some of the Titus styles were extreme, like this full close crop with only a tiny border of tendrils to frame the face. ('Costumes Parisiens', 1801)

the Titus first appeared in the aftermath of the Terror as a style worn by '*les Incroyables*', a group of daring young fashionistas who used fashion as protest.

D. Rothe De Nugent wrote a booklet of 1813 *Anti Titus Ou Remarques Critiques Sur La Coiffure Des Femmes Au Xix Siecle ...* lamenting how women had embraced this unfeminine style. He said that he found the style profoundly disgusting as it made women look as though they had Roman male heads on their female bodies. Conversely, in praise of the Titus, *Eloge de la Coiffure a la Titus*, written in 1810 by the French hairdresser Palette, said that the Titus was: 'the prettiest, the most agreeable, the most flirtatious style that has appeared since the beginning of the world'. He also commended it to his intended audience of fellow hairdressing professionals: 'women need to have haircuts, which their chambermaids can't do for them; and for occasions when they want fancier styles, they need "cache-folies" the false hairpieces which hairdressers would also provide'.

Although many women made the crop, few kept it for long. Maybe it was fear of disapproval impacting on marriageability, or maybe it was the desire for fashionable change. Wigs and hairpieces brought the magic of quick change without commitment and many women chose to wear their natural hair short during the day and have the versatility of a fashionable wig for evening occasions which amply aided the post-crop transition.

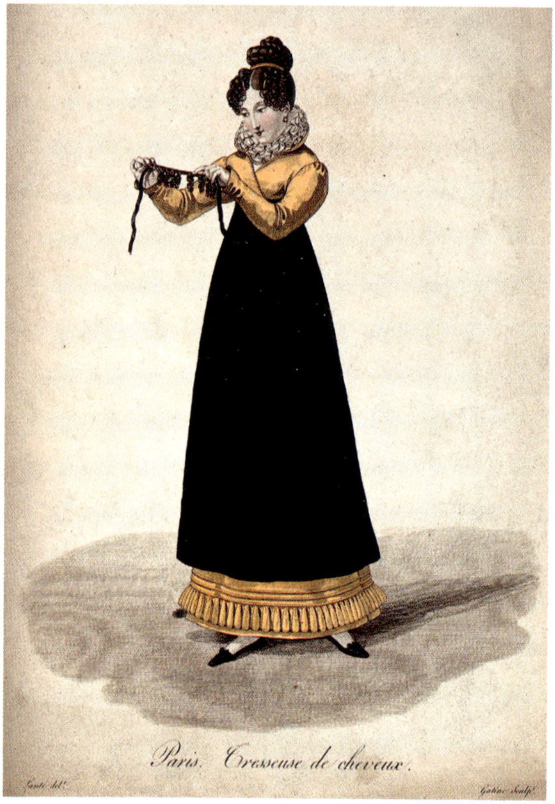

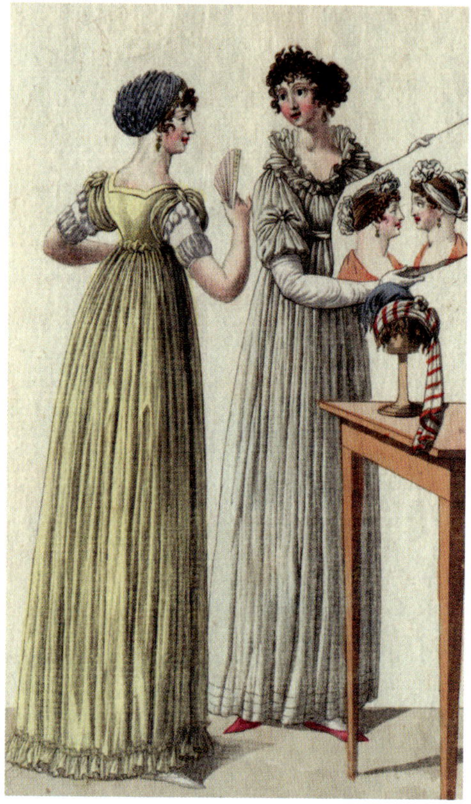

Above left: Cresseuse de Cheveaux, a Parisien maker of *cache-folies, c.* 1810. The ribbon of ringlets could be tied to give a fall of ringlets at the back of the neck, or around a chignon to add volume.

Above right: Millinery fashion plate, *Neues Journal Fur Fabrik*, 1809. On the wig stand is a bandeau headdress with a fringe of artificial hair attached.

By 1813 the *Coiffure a la Chinoise* came to the fore, with a stack of curls in front of a bun high on the crown of the head. It was a style that the novelist George Sand had worn in her youth, complaining bitterly in her autobiography that:

> besides its ugliness it was torture to have one's hair pulled the wrong way. It took a week of intense pain and insomnia before the hair took the right shape; and to force it into it, they put bands around the head so tightly that the skin of one's forehead was pulled up, and the sides of the eyes were lifted making one look like figures on a Chinese fan.

In *Northanger Abbey* Catherine has her hair 'cut and dressed by the best hand' before attending her first assembly in the Upper Rooms at Bath. At age fifteen she had 'began to curl her hair and long for balls' so it was inevitable that she would find a fine hairdresser in the fashionable city.

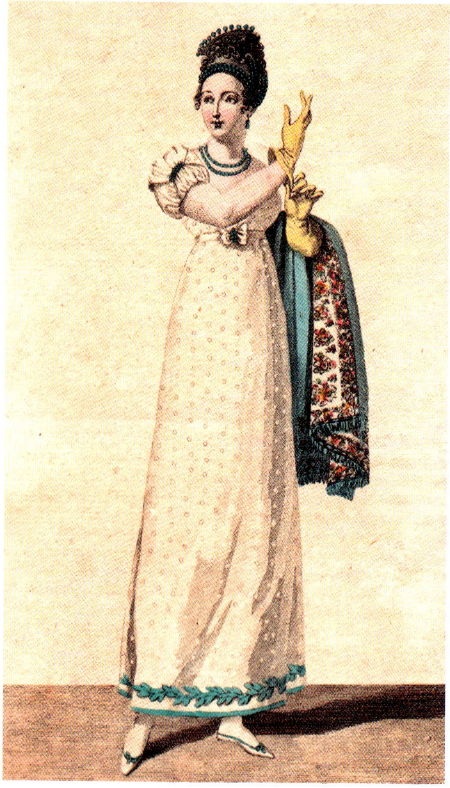

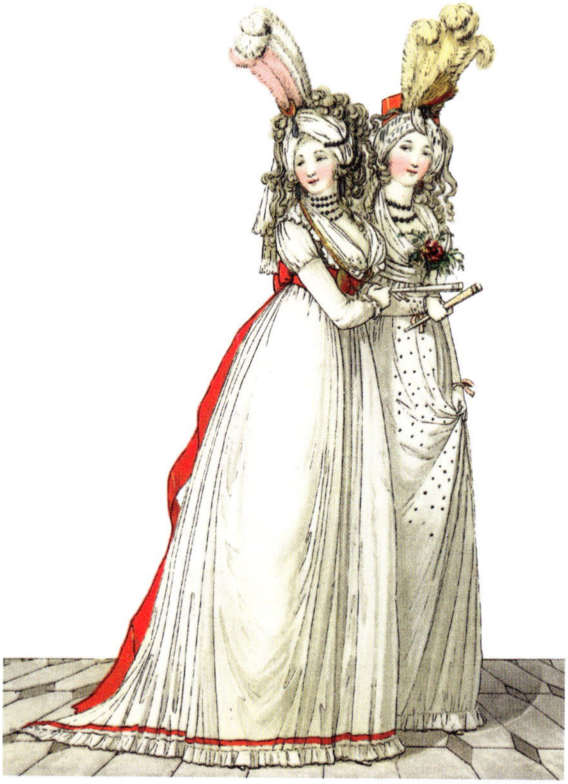

Above left: 'Coiffure à la Chinoise', 'Costumes Parisien', 1813.

Above right: Heideloff's 'Gallery of Fashion', 1795. In *Northanger Abbey*, as Catherine and Mrs Allen negotiated their way across the crowded ballroom, 'they saw nothing of the dancers but the high feathers of some of the ladies'.

When they meet at the theatre Isabella says to Catherine: 'you really have done your hair in a more heavenly style than ever: you mischievous creature, do you want to attract every body? I assure you, my brother is quite in love with you already'.

Catherine dreams of being a fine heroine like those in her favourite gothic novels, but unfortunately as she is healthy with both parents alive, and has no nefarious secrets languishing in the family closet, she is ill qualified. She doesn't have the looks either, a heroine is always heartbreakingly beautiful, but sadly Catherine is plain. Jane describes her:

> Catherine for many years of her life [was] as plain as any. She had a thin awkward figure, a sallow skin without colour, and strong features ... at fifteen appearances were mending; 'Catherine grows quite a good-looking girl, – she is almost pretty to-day' were words which caught her ears now and then; and how welcome were the sounds! To look almost pretty is an acquisition of higher delight to a girl who has been looking plain the first fifteen years of her life, than a beauty from her cradle can ever receive.

The importance of curls is reinforced when Isabella 'having gone through the usual ceremonial of meeting her friend with the most smiling affectionate haste, of admiring the set of her gown and envying the curl of her hair', only then could they happily 'follow their chaperone's arm in arm into the ballroom'.

It would be fascinating to know how Catherine resolved the problem of her lank hair – did she purchase a *'cache-folie'* to add to her hair, or did the hairdresser introduce her to:

> ATKINSON's CURLING FLUID,
> Well known for its singular efficacy in restoring the hair where it has fallen off from illness, perspiration, change of climate, &c. It is also much esteemed by ladies for making the hair beautifully soft and glossy, and for preserving it in curl during exercise in dancing or walking, or in damp weather.

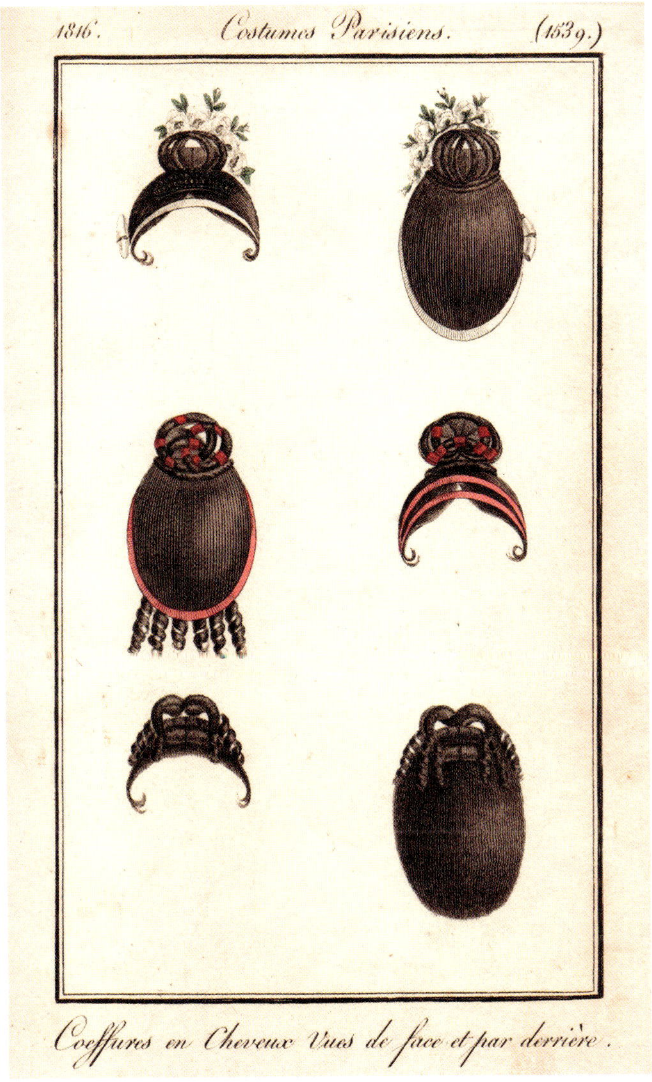
1816.
Costumes Parisiens.
(1539.)
Coeffures en Cheveux Vues de face et par derrière.

Left: Coiffures from 'Costumes Parisiens', 1816.

Opposite: *London Evening Dresses*, printed for Richard Phillips in January 1804.

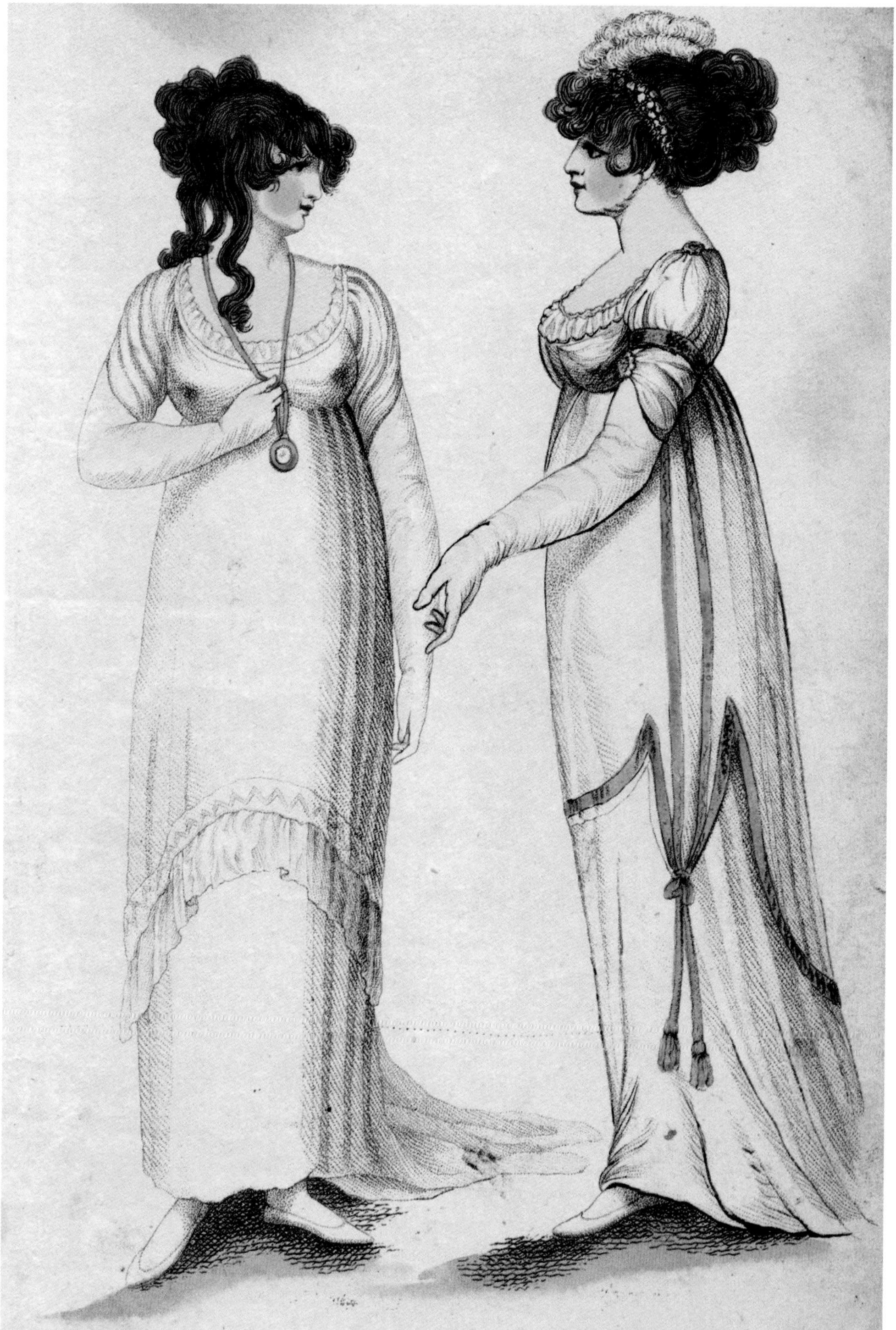

LONDON EVENING DRESES.

Printed for RICHARD PHILLIPS, N° 71, St. Paul's Church Yard.

While staying at glamorous Godmersham Park, in a letter to Cassandra dated Saturday 24 August 1805, Jane wrote about the visiting hairdresser:

> Mr. Hall walked off this morning to Ospringe, with no inconsiderable booty. He charged Elizabeth 5s. for every time of dressing her hair, and 5s. for every lesson to Sace, allowing nothing for the pleasures of his visit here, for meat, drink, and lodging, the benefit of country air, and the charms of Mrs. Salkeld's and Mrs. Sace's society. Towards me he was as considerate as I had hoped for from my relationship to you, charging me only 2s. 6d. for cutting my hair, though it was as thoroughly dressed after being cut for Eastwell as it had been for the Ashford assembly. He certainly respects either our youth or our poverty.

Those lucky enough to live in fashionably large houses would have a dressing room often as a space between the husband and wife's individual bedrooms, while for those with less space, the dressing table was an increasingly fashionable piece of furniture. For a healthy budget, Sheraton's beautiful creations were much in demand. For a more modest budget there were delightful table-top standing mirrors that could be angled, usually with a couple of lockable drawers below so that – as Jane did in Southampton – an old table could be repurposed as a dressing table.

In February 1807 Jane wrote from Southampton about home improvements including their new dressing table:

> Our dressing table is constructing on the spot, out of a large kitchen table belonging to the house, for doing which we have the permission of Mr. Husket, Lord Lansdown's painter – domestic painter, I should call him, and I suppose whenever the walls want no touching up he is employed about my lady's face.

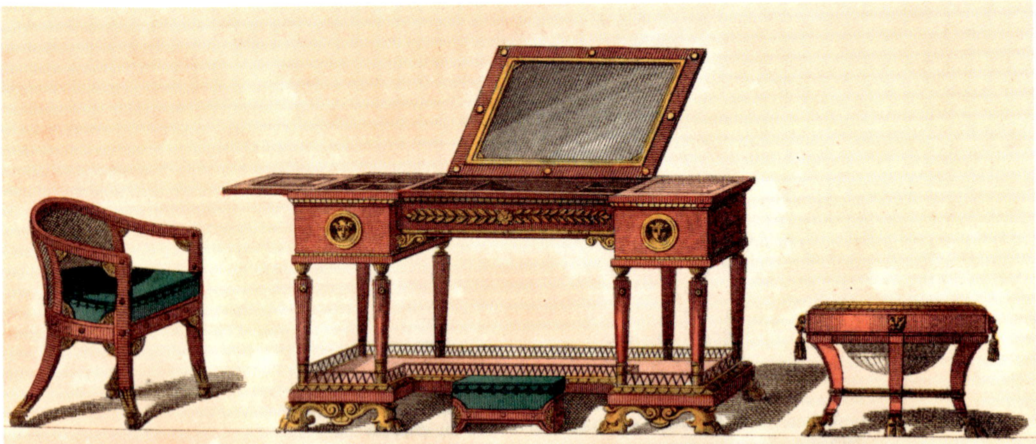

'Ladies Toilet Fauteuil, and Chamber Bath', Ackermann's *Repository of Arts*, 1809. The dressing table has multiple compartments for 'every requisite of the accomplished female'. The chamber bath, a wide basin on a low stand (to the right), was described as 'the most proper article for the promotion of health.

6

The Dandy Barber

The modern man was modelled after military heroes such as Nelson and Wellington, and many military uniforms were very flamboyant promoting an idealised masculinity. Just as the statuary of the ancient world was the inspiration for feminine beauty, the heroic proportions of classical statues informed the male ideal. They also often showed them unclothed, so naturally a trouser to define a strong well-turned leg would be bias cut and skin tight in a light neutral shade almost the colour of flesh. For those with less than

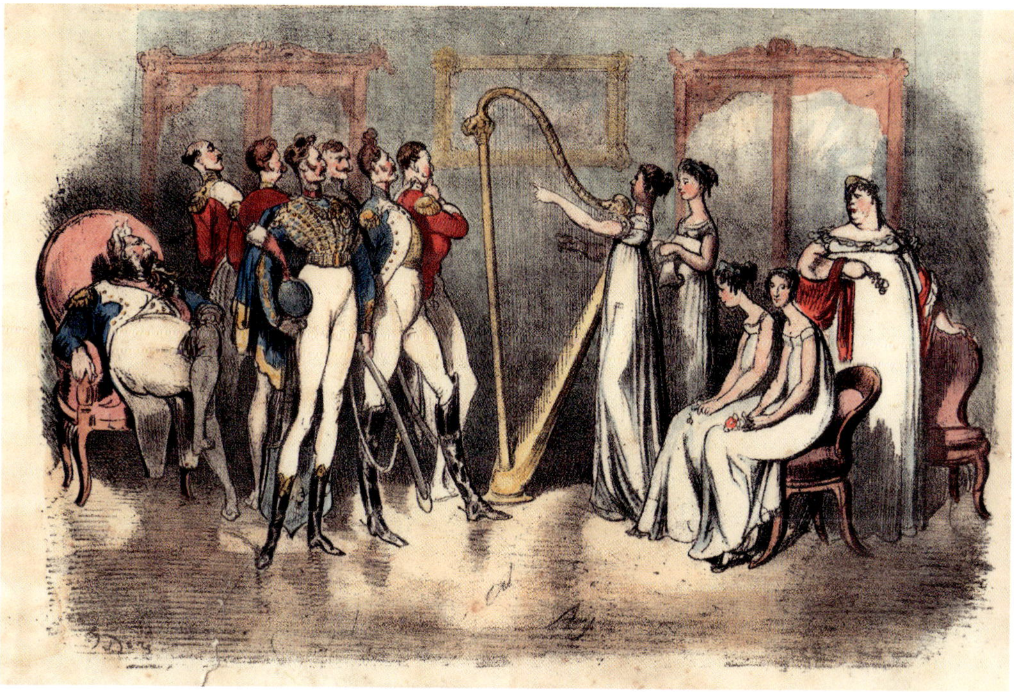

'Musical Entertainments', *c.* 1800. Under the watchful eye of her stout mother, the harpist plays to impress their swaggering military guests, while her sisters barely conceal their boredom.

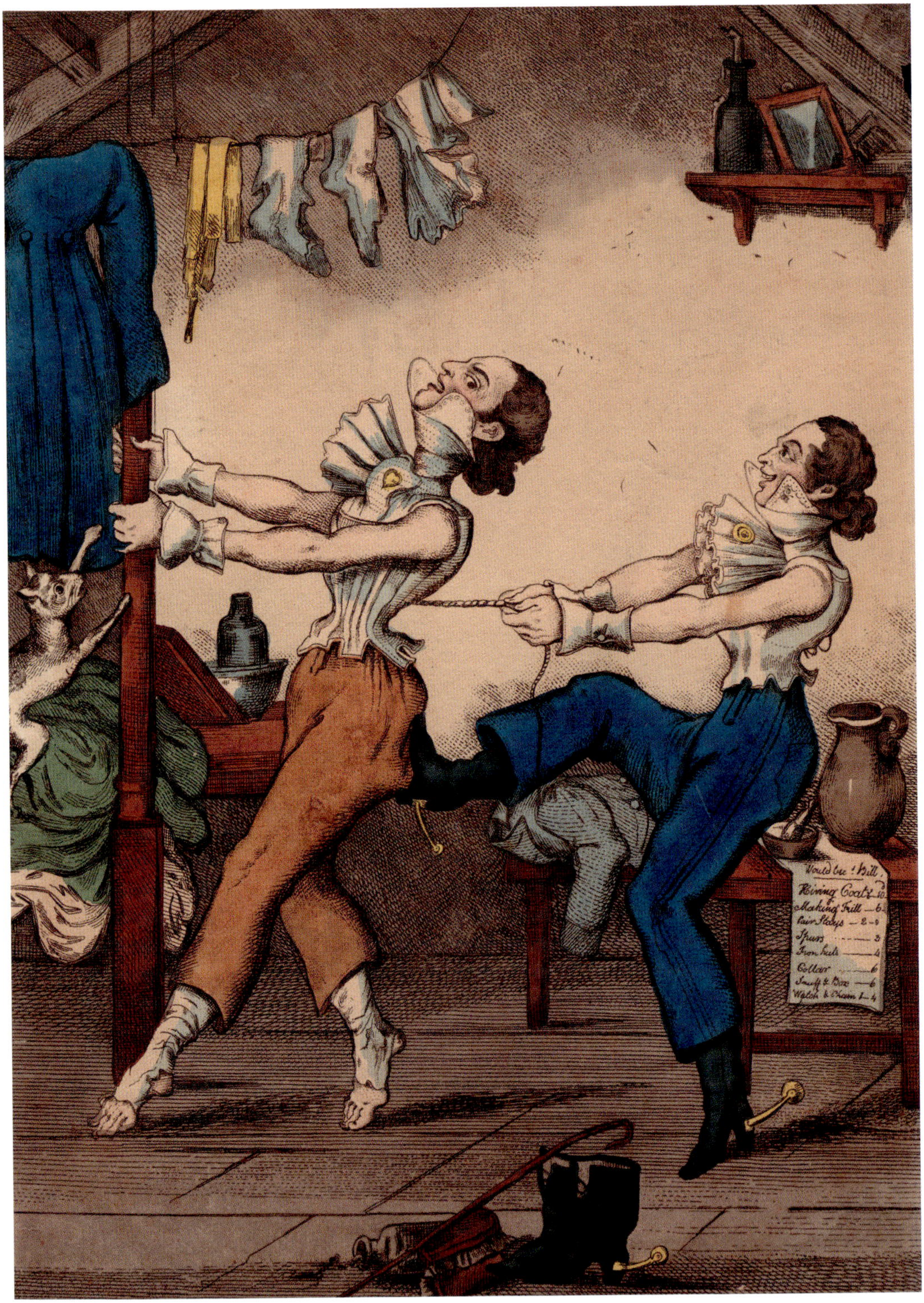
Would be ! Bill
Hiring Coat £10
Making Frill — 6
Pair Stays — 2–0
Spurs —— 3
Iron heels —— 4
Collar —— 6
Snuff & Box — 6
Watch & Chain 1–4

A satirical drawing of one dandy tightly lacing another into his Brummell bodice to give him the desired tiny torso.

heroic proportions, the art of the tailor sculpted them anew from cloth, padding scrawny shoulders and arms, puffing out sunken chests and rendering puny legs more 'poetic' by judicious padding and false calves. As in the Elizabethan era, good legs were particularly important not just to fill out the fashionable trouser or pantalon, but as an indicator of well-practiced skills at fencing and horsemanship.

Like Willoughby, Wickham was a handsome man poised to take full advantage of his looks and the assurance of his military swagger, and as soon as Kitty and Lydia spot him they are dying to know everything about him as: 'His appearance was greatly in his favour: he had all the best parts of beauty, a fine countenance, a good figure, and very pleasing address. [He] wanted only regimentals to make him completely charming.'

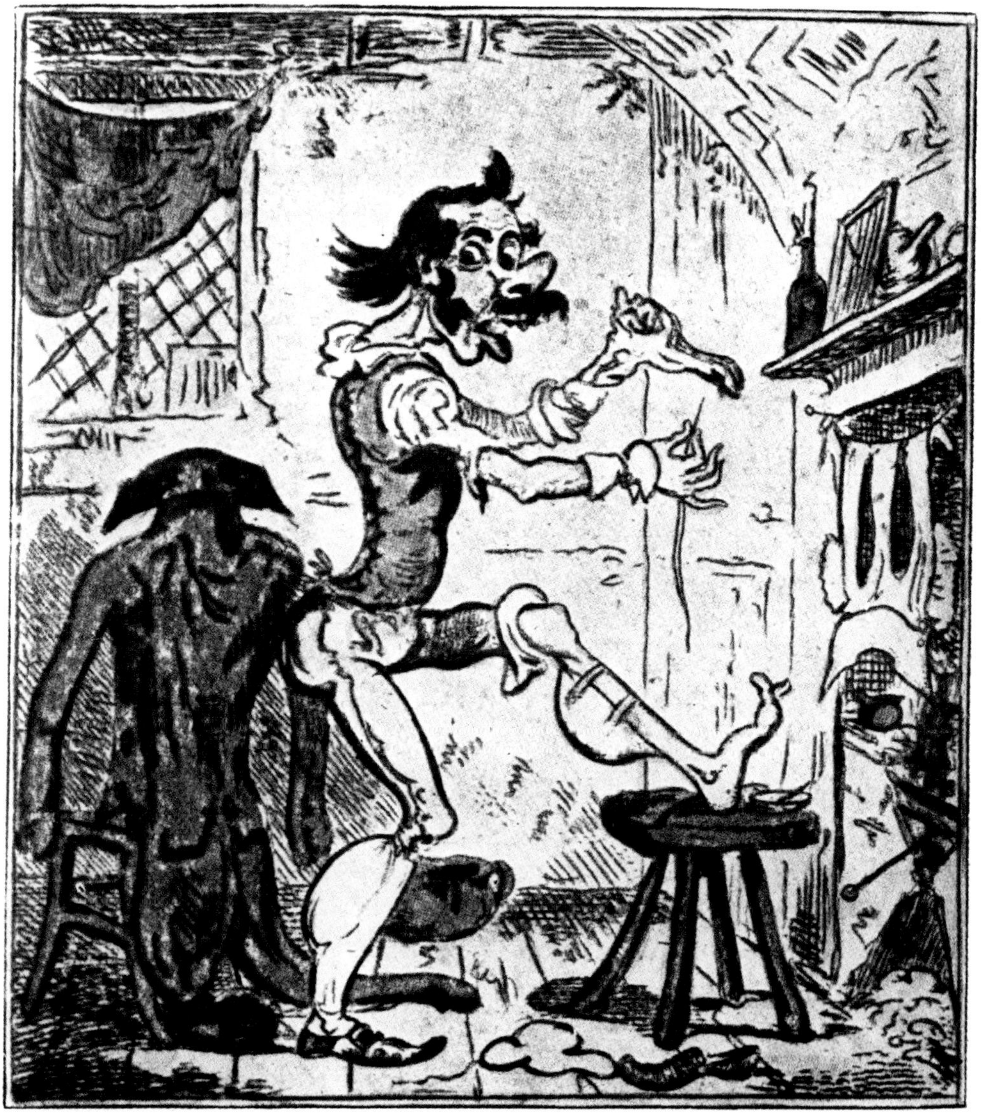

'A Gentleman's Toilet' (Lewis Marks, 1800), a caricature of false calves.

It was not surprising that all the girls – and women – liked a man in uniform because most regiments actually selected their recruits for their tall, slim stature and youthful good looks. Some colonels actually found reason to discharge their veteran officers despite their obvious value in the melee because they wanted to replace them with younger, more attractive men to improve the look of their regiment and therefore its prestige.

The early nineteenth-century dandy was as much a narcissist as his foppish eighteenth-century predecessor, but instead of gratifying his vanity by adding pomade and powder, he took pride in shaving every hair to perfection and buffing and polishing his complexion to abject cleanliness. Just as there were instruction manuals for young women, books such as *The Whole Art of Dress* written by 'a Cavalry Officer' offered advice on personal grooming and presentation.

In an age where hot water was not on tap, he reminds his readers to organise warm water for washing face and hands: in 'both summer and winter' for 'its efficacy in opening the pores of the skin, which is softened, refreshed, and refined by its application .... In winter, indeed, it is the only way of thoroughly cleansing the skin.'

In the choice of soap for the complexion he advises to avoid use of common yellow soap unless 'a skin dry and shining, like polished brass, be desired'. For those wrinkled unfortunates like Admiral Baldwin, instead of preparations like Gowland's lotion he recommends: 'the use of fine Scotch oatmeal, which possesses a peculiar property of whitening the skin and rendering it very soft, whether face or hands'. If only Admiral Baldwin had known! He could also have used it for his hands, as the Cavalry Officer assures that it is very efficacious as he, and a number of his friends have been able to restore their hands to the correct colour and texture of those of a gentleman.

He also gives instructions for the fingernails which are much like those Regency women used for their manicures. He writes: 'Of the nails, which form the most important portion of the hand, if thin, they should be scraped until they obtain a sufficient thickness, this paring

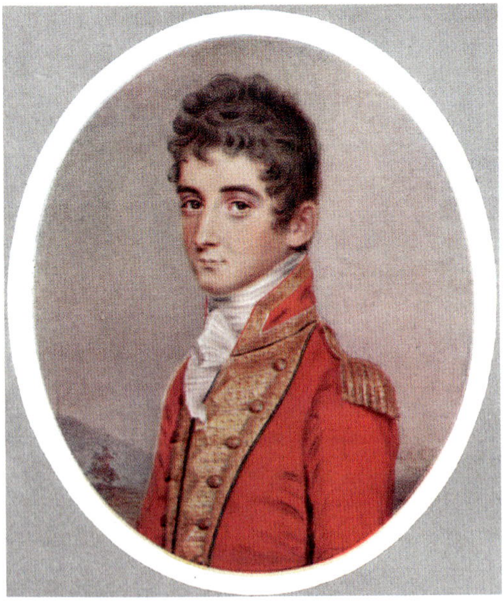

Lieutenant Lygon (portrait miniature by John Smart Jr, 1803). A handsome officer with carefully curled hair brought forward onto his forehead in a Titus style.

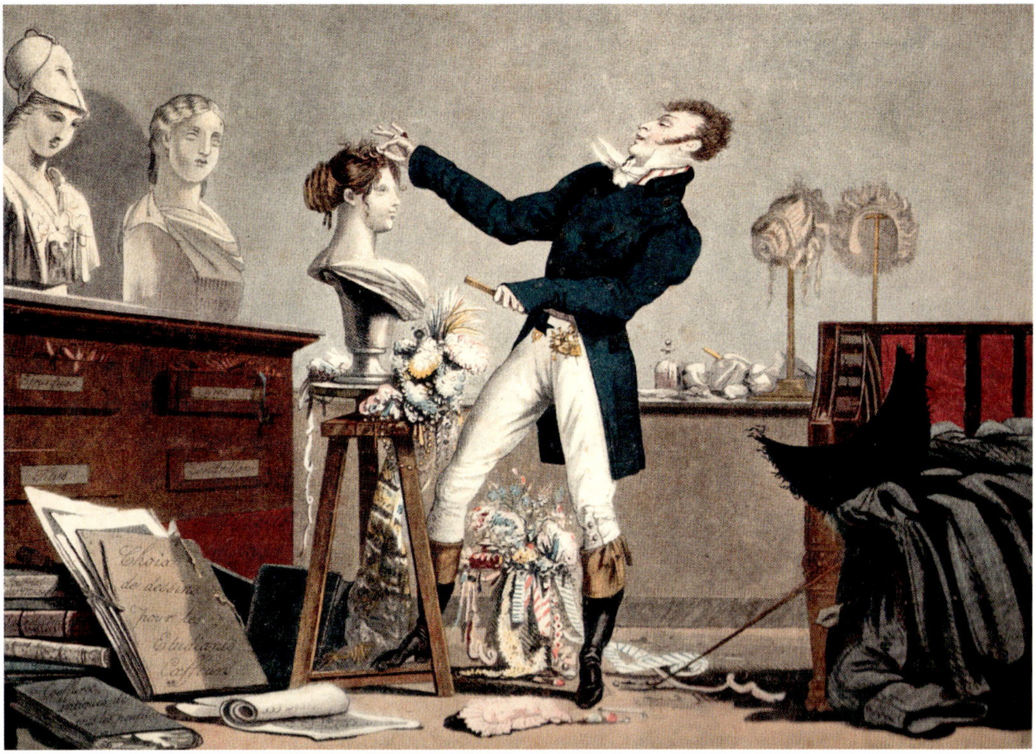

'The Dandy Barber'. The exquisitely styled hairdresser is creating wigs and hairpieces modelled on classical statuary.

likewise gives them a good colour and gloss ... Filbert-nails are the most approved for beauty', advising that this shape can be obtained by habitually after washing in hot water 'turning the skin that skirts them back with the towel, when the nail will appear much longer, and more filbert-like than it would otherwise have done'. However, the Dandy would go further in his pursuit of a fine gentlemanly hand, applying white wax to the underside of the nails.

Throughout the eighteenth century wigs and powder had protected men from any prejudice against premature greying or baldness as their natural hair was never seen, but with the change of fashion provoked by the Hair Powder Tax of 1795, hair became as important to men as it was to women. This became very clear to Jane when, to her amusement and that of her family, her midshipman brother Charles arrived sporting cropped hair free from powder when he paid a brief visit home before playing his heroic part in the capture of the *Scipio c.* 1801. Although purportedly cropped short for convenience on board ship, it happily coincided with the change in fashion despite the general reluctance of the Navy to update uniform regulations.

Frank Churchill's hair features in the plot of *Emma*:

> Emma's very good opinion of Frank Churchill was a little shaken the following day, by hearing that he was gone off to London, merely to have his hair cut ... There was certainly no harm in his travelling sixteen miles twice over on such an errand; but there was an air of foppery and nonsense in it which she could not approve.

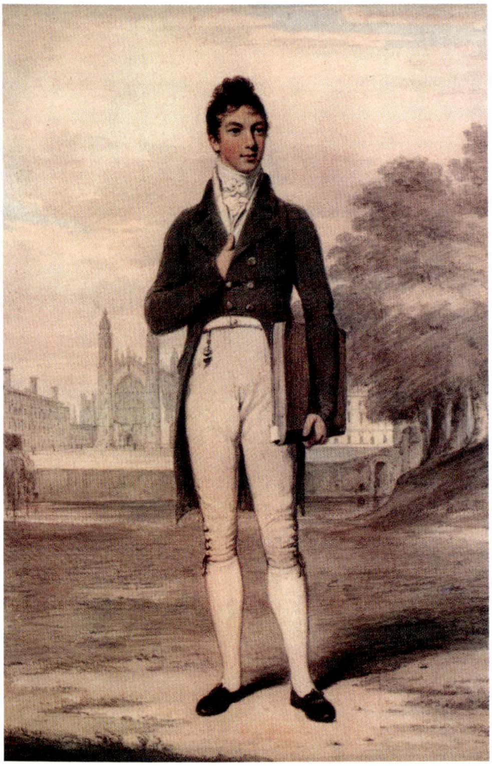 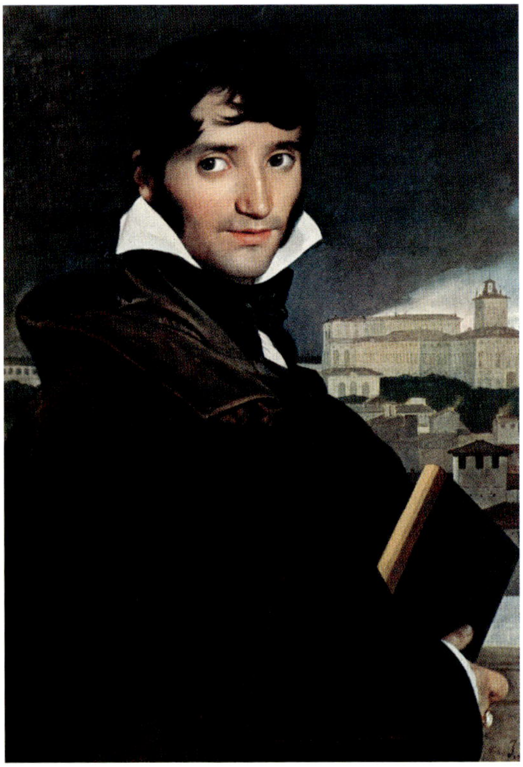

Above left: Revd Henry Mortlock (Henry Edridge ARA). He wears a fashionable Titus hairstyle, *c.* 1809.

Above right: The lush sideburns of the artist François Marius Granet (Jean-Auguste-Dominique Ingres, 1807).

Emma is concerned that it is indicative of his vanity and his lack of consideration to take such a huge amount of time for himself during a short visit. Had it not been a device to conceal his secret purchase of the pianoforte for his secret fiancée Jane Fairfax, a trip to the capital to have the best possible haircut still might have been warranted. The cropped Titus style for men as well as women demanded a good cut to encourage just the correct multidirectional curl falling gracefully from the crown in the style of an eminent Roman. The cropped styles, sometimes very short, often with a soft curl over the forehead or brought forward to frame the face – and frequently a combination of both – allowed for the introduction of side whiskers. Early incarnations at the turn of the century were usually very precisely formed sideburns closely trimmed and guided straight down to frame the jaw line, but after 1810 it became popular to trim them at a careful diagonal to enhance the cheekbones.

The author of *The Whole Art of Dress* asserts that as the hair 'has such capabilities for setting off the most indifferent countenance' it is of significant importance and should be carefully cared for: 'The chief attributes of hair should be curl, strength, and gloss, all three of which, art can make up.' Hair should be oiled every morning to nourish it, with Bear's

Grease or Macassar oil applied at the root and rubbed in well using alternately 'A hard penetrating, and a soft brush ... The former strengthens the roots of the hair by impelling a brisker circulation of the blood, while the latter bestows the shine or polish.' It should be washed once a fortnight in summer and once a month in winter and trimmed once a month, 'as it seems to fade and droop, and the ends split'.

Those disenchanted with Bear's Grease or Macassar oil could try one of the first commercial shampoos. An advertisement in Ackermann's *Repository of Arts* for December 1809 offered:

> THE ONLY HAIR-WASH IN ENGLAND.
> ROYAL BRITISH ARCANUM, It not only promotes the growth [of hair], it prevents it from turning grey, or falling off ... rendering it extremely glossy, soft, and beautiful; in fact, no one who wishes to possess a good and clean head of hair, will fail using it once or twice a week.

Even more interesting are the extravagant health benefits, claiming that it will prevent headache and sight loss.

Sadly, it is not recorded if Beau Brummell ever used Royal British Arcanum, but it is likely that the idea of a specialist hair-wash would have appealed to him. Captain William Jesse reports in his *Life of George Brummel Esq* that he was in attendance one day for Brummel's toilette, posted safely in an anteroom where Beau Brummell thought he was out of sight. He no doubt would have been horrified to know that Jesse was secretly able to

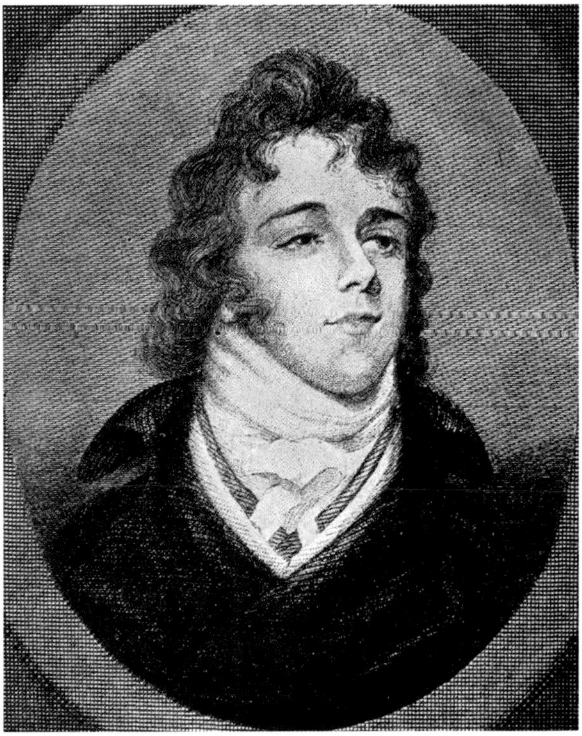

Beau Brummell as a young man with elegant sideburns (engraved by J. Cooke).

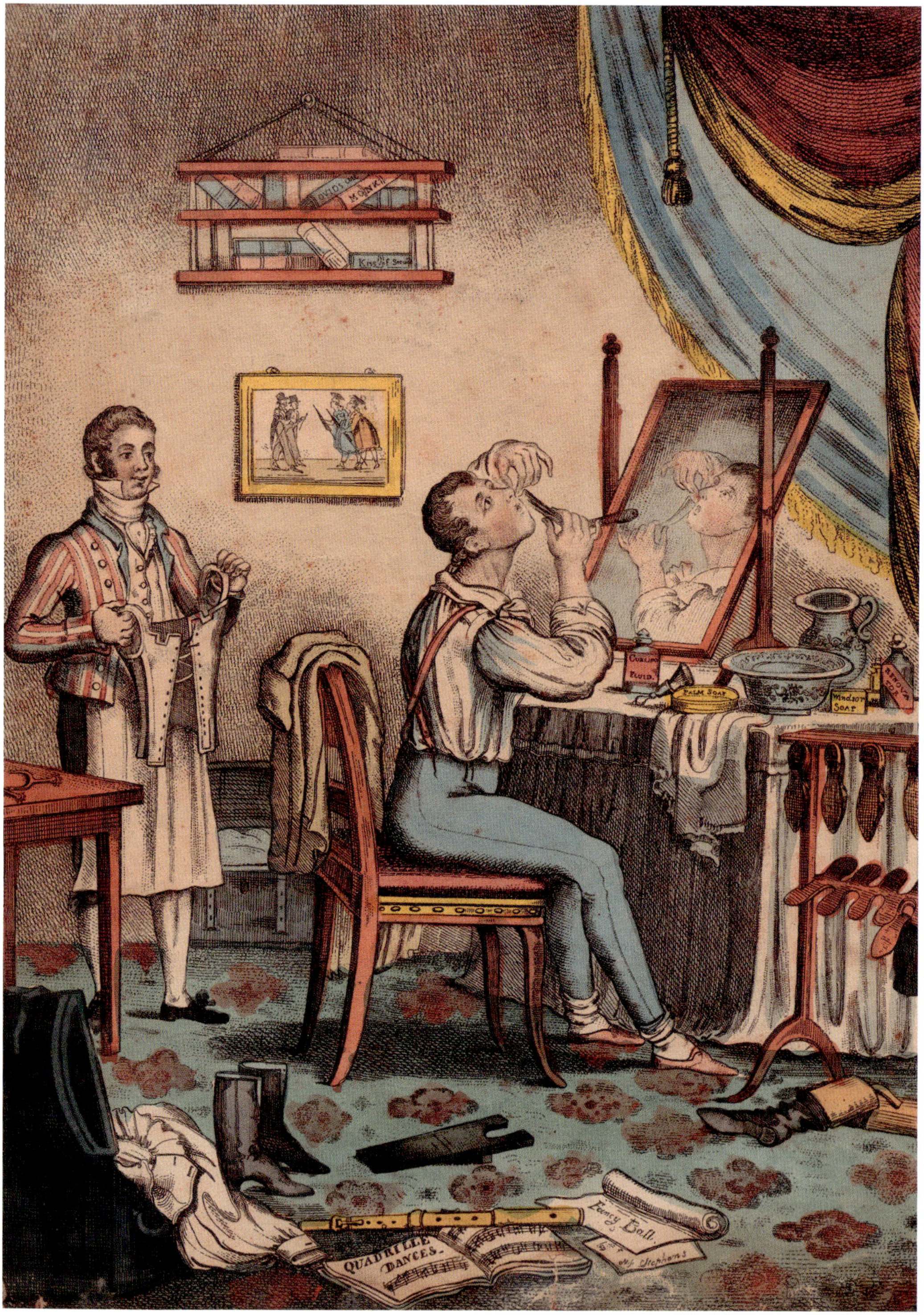

A satirical drawing of a dandy shaving himself to perfection as exemplified by Beau Brummell. He has a bar of transparent palm soap and a bottle of curling fluid on his dressing table.

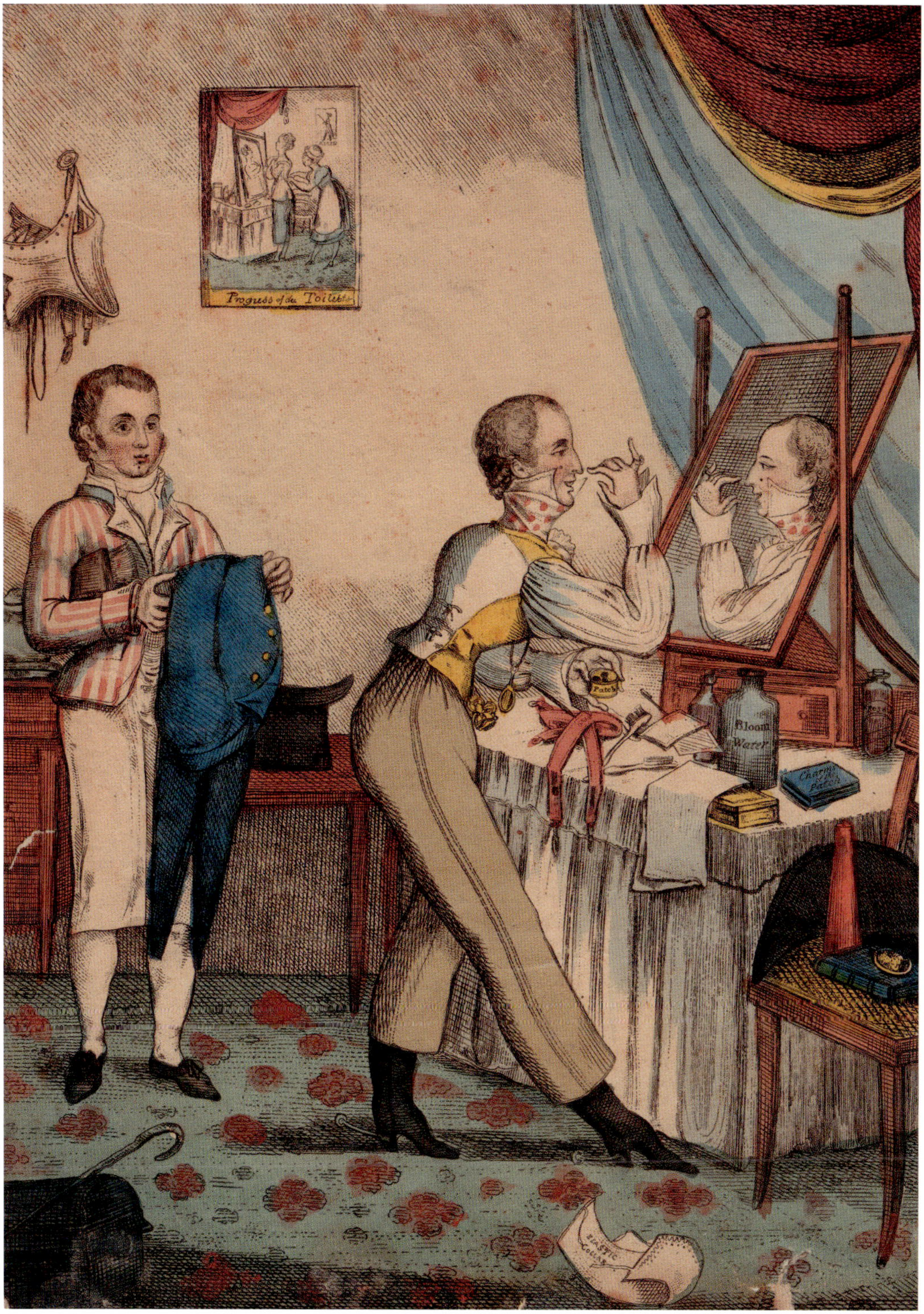

A satirical drawing of a dandy adding patches as the 'final touch'. He has bottles of Bloom Water and Milk of Roses on his dressing table.

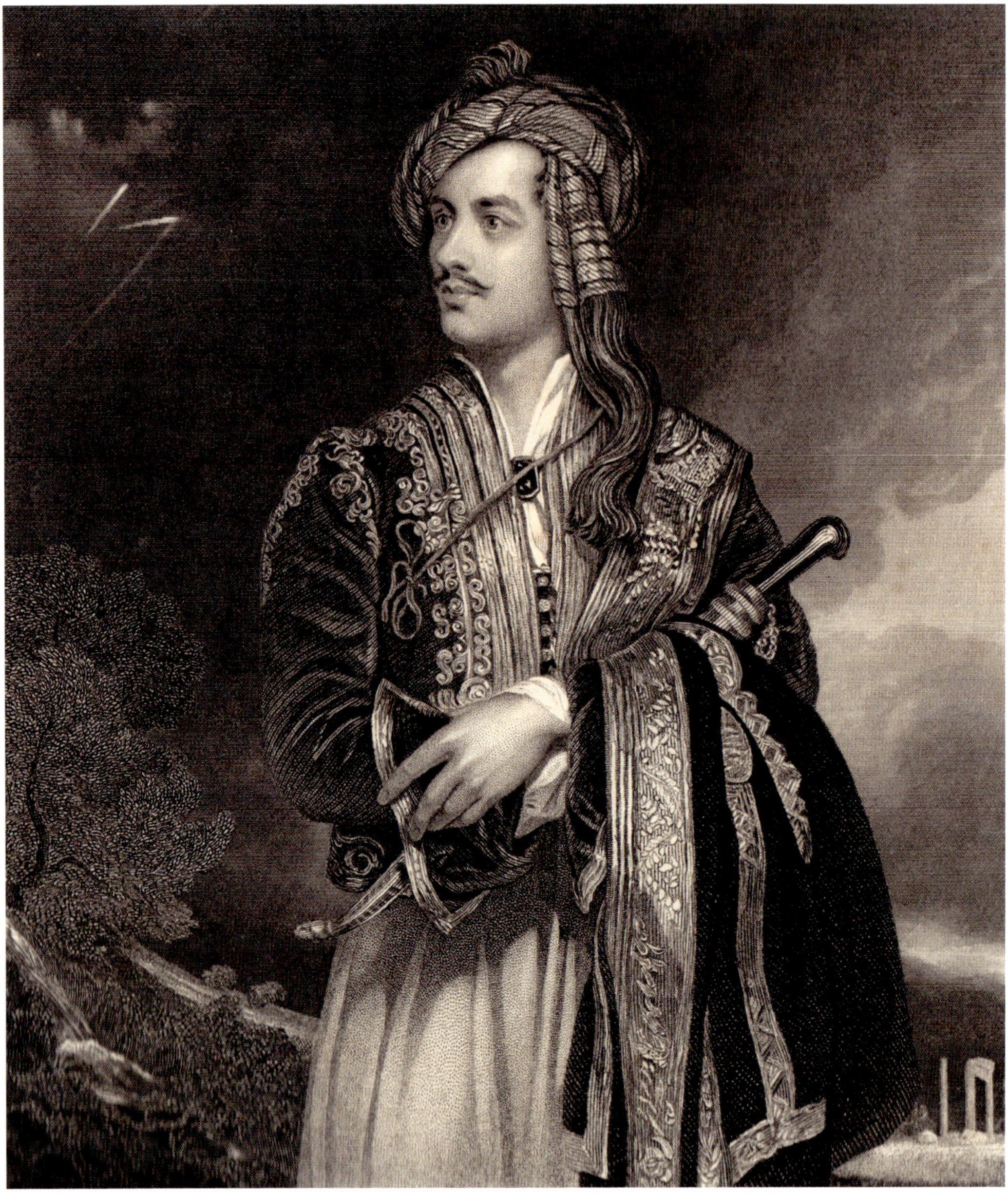

'Lord Byron in Albanian Dress' (after Thomas Phillips, 1813). The handsome poet was said to wear curling papers to bed and to be as vain of his curls as a girl of sixteen.

catch a full view of him reflected in the mirror without his wig and naked whilst he used his flesh brush all over. He reported:

> The Beau took a dentist's mirror in one hand, and a pair of tweezers in the other, and thus nobly armed, closely scanned his forehead and well-shaved chin, and did not lay

> them down till he had drawn, with a resolution and perseverance truly extraordinary, and totally regardless of the exquisite pain the removal of each elegant extract must have caused him every stray hair that could be detected on the surface of his venerable mug!

He still spent at least two hours each day in grooming, and it was the loss of this routine – as well as the execrable food – that caused him the most distress when he was sentenced to The Prison Royale, a French debtor's prison in 1835. He was deeply distressed by the absence of his: 'jug and basin, his dentist's mirror, his tweezers, and his silver shaving and expectorating dish, his toilette, his soaps, pommades, and eau de Cologne', and found it impossible to adjust until his friends managed to restore them to him. Whilst there, he struck up a relationship with Charles Godefroi, the editor of the *Ami de la Verité* who was held for his political beliefs. Godefroi was more than surprised by his grooming regimen, seemingly astonished as much by the fact that 'he actually washed and shaved every day' as the three hours he took each day to do it.

Lord Byron once wrote of Beau Brummell as having nothing remarkable in his style of dress, except a 'certain exquisite propriety', and Jane could have written much the same for Darcy. She describes Mr Bingley as 'good-looking and gentlemanlike: he had a pleasant countenance, and easy, unaffected manners', but Darcy she leaves as something of an enigma: 'Mr. Darcy, soon drew the attention of the room by his fine, tall person, handsome features, noble mien.' She makes it clear that his looks are enhanced to many by his ten thousand a year, to which: 'The gentlemen pronounced him to be a fine figure of a man, the ladies declared he was much handsomer than Mr. Bingley'. However, for Jane, and for Lizzie, it is his clear countenance capable of emotion that is his chief attraction and several times it is noted that his colour changes according to his emotions. This shows him to be genuine, and is just as attractive a quality for a gentleman as it is for a lady.

7

Beauty in Nature

The tall, the graceful, the lithe and the young were almost all delighted to be granted the freedom of a slender silhouette unencumbered by hoop or heels. But for many women plumped by a lifetime of pregnancy or Georgian fine dining, the obligation to attain a slender natural figure without the support of stays was too much. The satirists had a field day at the expense of the short, the stout and the ungainly as women were forced on a journey of self-loathing that continues until this day.

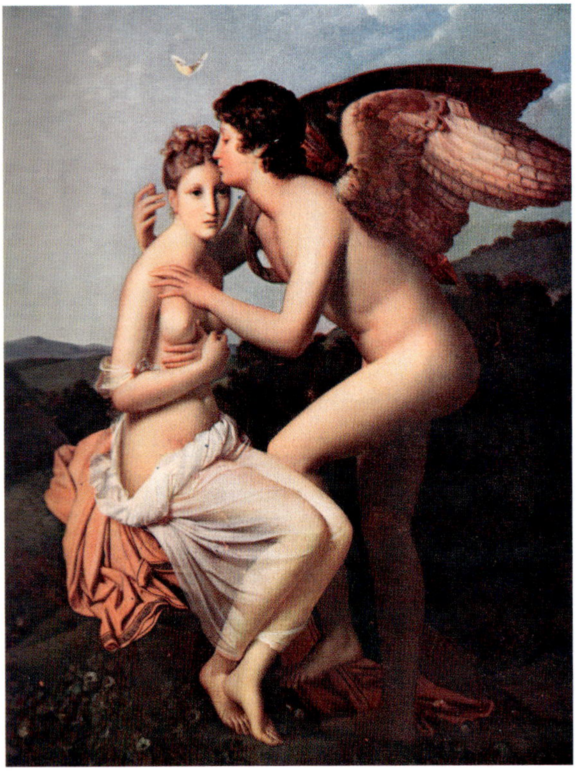

Cupid and Psyche (François Gérard, 1798). This was exhibited in 1798 and became the contemporary beauty ideal. Everyone wanted to have such a fine figure and perfect, luminous complexion.

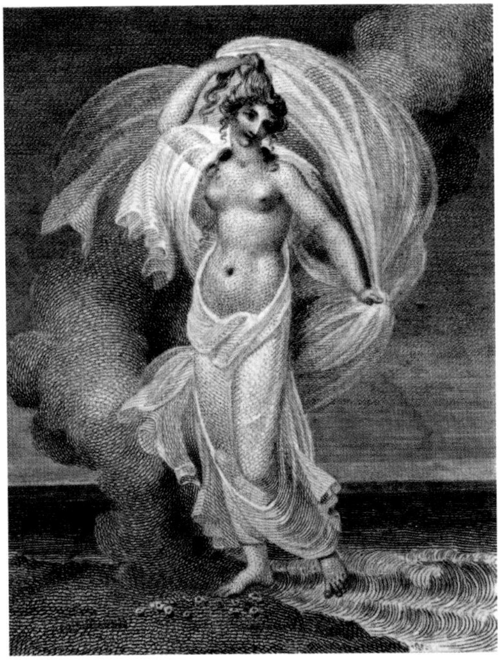

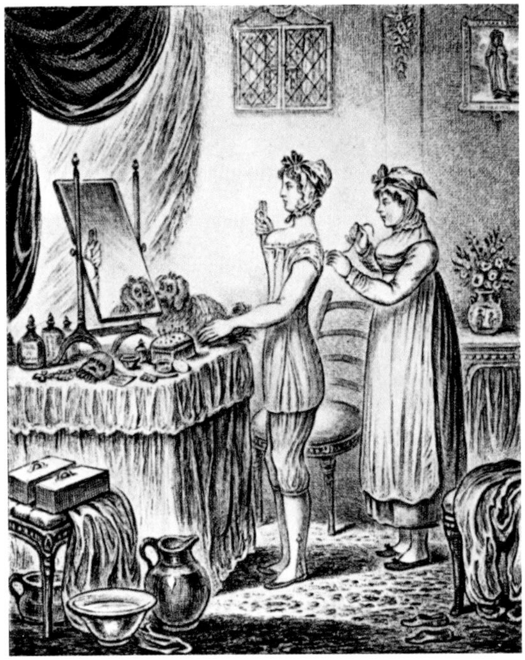

Above left: *The Birth of Venus*, 1811.

Above right: 'The Stays' from 'The Progress of the Toilet' series, James Gillray, 1810.

The gorgeous form of the Grecian goddess in all her marble splendour became the new body ideal, from her long slender neck to her high bosom and willowy limbs. The majority of statuary was formed to display the delicate folds and drapery of the classical gown that was cinched only with a narrow sash or filet beneath the bosom. This inspired the Neoclassical high-waisted gown that became the fashion for the first two decades of the nineteenth century and necessitated a new set of underpinnings.

The 'three graces', Juliette Récamier, Térézia Tallien and Josephine Buonaparte, had scandalised Paris with their daringly sheer gowns worn without stays – or as it was rumoured, anything at all – but for the majority, stays simply changed shape and emphasis. Traditional corsetry had focussed on perfecting the hourglass and pushing the bosoms up and together whilst trimming the waist, but the new styles for stays either concentrated on slimming the hips to little more than the size of the waist, or were short, centred only on the bust.

Although in Paris the high-waisted silhouette was lauded as the apex of the refinement of classical antiquity, in Britain the waist-less gown was initially greeted as an abomination especially by male commentators as in the satirical song 'Shepherds, I Have Lost My Waist':

Shepherds, I have lost my waist,
Have you seen my body?
Sacrificed to modern taste,
I'm quite a hoddy-doddy!

For fashion I that part forsook
Where sages place the belly;
'Tis gone – and I have not a nook
For cheesecake, tart or jelly.

What was very apparent to all viewers of ancient statuary was that the bust was formed with each pert round breast clearly and separately defined, unlike the conjoined bust that traditional stays produced. Featured in many fashion plates, this entirely new emphasis inspired the 'divorce', a punning name for a new corset that kept the breasts separate and according to *The Mirror of the Graces* in 1811 'it consists of a piece of steel or iron of triangular form, gently curved on each side. This formidable breast-plate (for the attraction of love's arrows not to repel them!) is covered with soft materials; and thus bedded, placed in the centre of the chest to divide the breasts ....'. It might have been to this that Jane referred in September 1813 when she wrote in a letter: 'the stays now are not made to force the bosom up at all; – that was a very unbecoming, unnatural fashion'.

The new emphasis on the bust created problems for those less well endowed, and the wax bosom was invented to create the illusion of fullness under a sheer bodice. The bosom friends had to be fitted to the individual, and a description in *The True Briton* in 1800 recorded how a father was horrified when returning home to find a very smart young

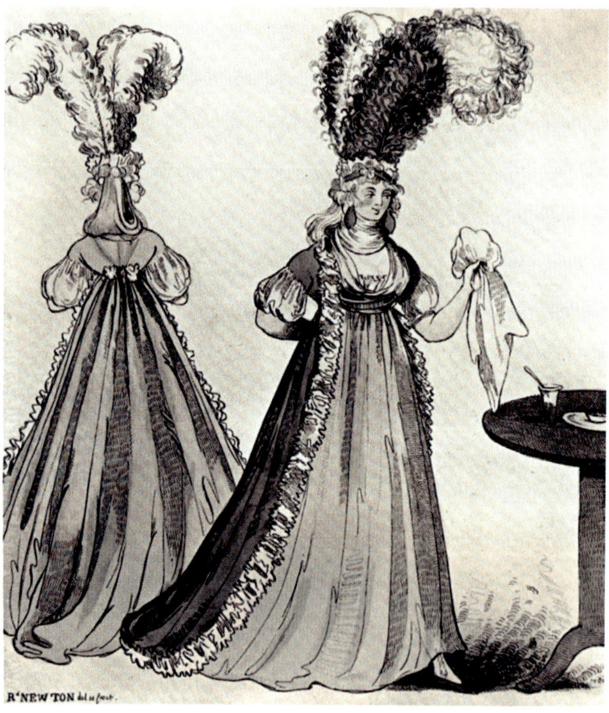

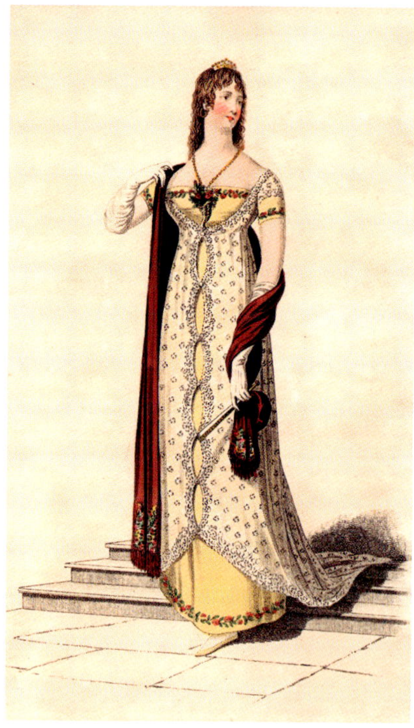

Above left: 'Shepherds, I have Lost My Waist' (Richard Newton, 1795).

Above right: 'Evening Visiting Dress', *La Belle Assemblée*, August 1810. It shows the wide-bosomed silhouette created by the Divorce corset.

man with his hands all over his fourteen-year-old daughter, only to be told by his wife 'the man is only fitting Euphrasia with a proper bosom; the girl cannot appear in fashionable company with her present horrid flatness of chest'.

To wax lyrical about wax bosoms: an epigram from *The Spirit of the Public Journals* of 1801:

WAXEN BOSOMS.
SPITE of the gibes of wanton wit,
What emblems can the fair,
Of their dear tender hearts more fit,
Than waxen bosoms wear?
'Twixt mounts of wax, and hills of snow,
How finall the difference felt!
With due degrees of heat we know
That both will gently melt.

There could however be far worse fates than a little melting as Mrs Ann Thicknesse related in her *School for Fashion* of 1801, a young lady and her betrothed were at a party that was so hot and overcrowded she fainted: 'the women eagerly flew to her assistance, and upon loosening her gown to give her more air, out tumbled a pair of beautiful wax breasts

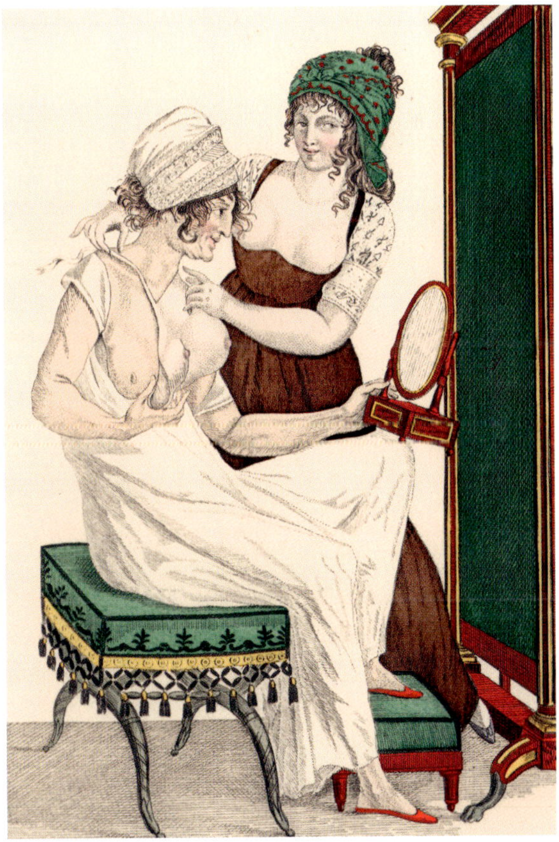

'La Toilette, Le Bon Genre', 1801.
An older lady being fitted for perky wax bosoms.

on the floor!! The ladies screamed, though we make no doubt but they secretly enjoyed this public discovery.' She then goes on to report with some relish that 'the disappointed lover; who had been without doubt so often fascinated with the beautiful snowy bosom of his mistress, which laid artfully half concealed under a transparent veil of gause ... was immediately filled by contempt and disgust!', adding the caution, 'Whilst women sport false bosoms, let them not complain of men possessing false hearts!'

Certainly, a fine bosom was to be esteemed and Regency gentlemen felt no compunction in admiring them even if it caused discomfort. In *Mansfield Park* Fanny arrives as a rather 'delicate and puny' ten-year-old and she has done her best to be unnoticeable ever since. Now in her late teens, to her mortification, she is admired widely when she wears her first 'grown-up' professionally made gown to a dinner party. Formal evening wear was décolleté and both Henry and Sir Thomas complement this new view of her, as Edmund tells her:

> Your uncle thinks you very pretty, dear Fanny ... Your complexion is so improved! – and you have gained so much countenance! – and your figure – nay, Fanny, do not turn away about it – it is but an uncle. If you cannot bear an uncle's admiration, what is to become of you? You must really begin to harden yourself to the idea of being worth looking at.

In many ways posture was even more important than a fine figure. Good posture, graceful movement and excellent deportment were the hallmarks of good breeding indicating a more aristocratic background. To be straight and upright indicated good character, polite manners, self-respect and self-control. Darcy has excellent posture as has Emma Woodhouse with her 'firm and upright figure'.

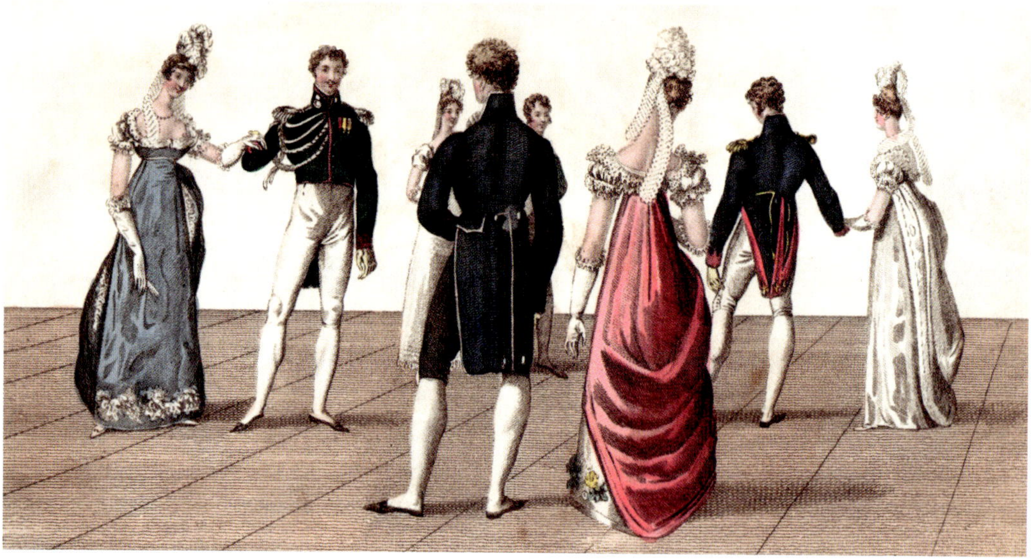

'Parisian Dancers No. 2 l'Horatia Quadrille', *La Belle Assemblée,* July 1820. Dancing helped to promote and maintain good posture – with so many onlookers, no one wanted to unclench their stomach muscles until they sat down.

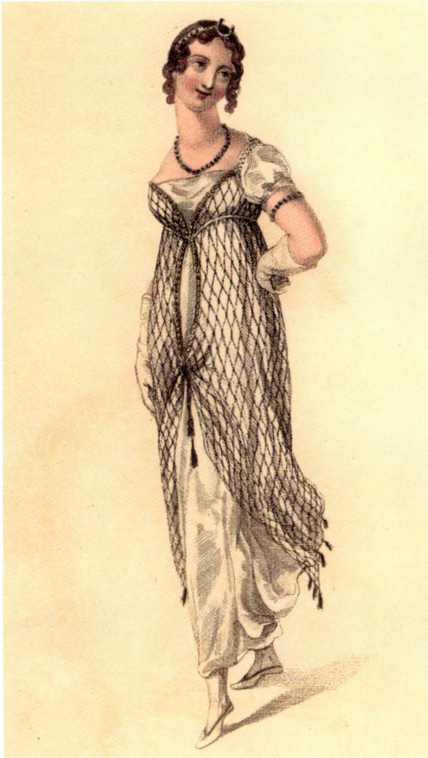

Right: 'Ball Dress', Ackermann's *Repository of Arts,* March 1810. A well-chosen ball gown would enhance graceful movements, drawing appreciative attention to the wearer.

Below: 'An Elegant Establishment for Young Ladies' (E. F. Burney, *c.* 1810). The Beauty School regime insisted that a girl not willing to work hard at developing beauty from within did not deserve beauty at all.

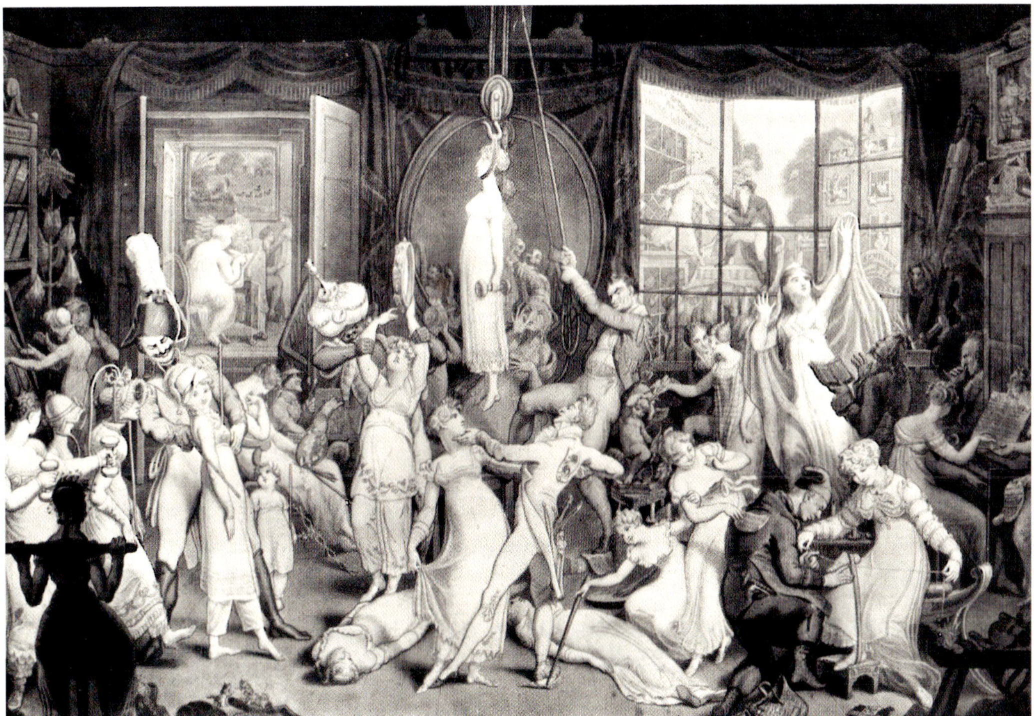

In *Pride and Prejudice* when Miss Bingley unexpectedly invites Lizzie to: 'take a turn about the room. I assure you it is very refreshing after sitting so long in one attitude.' Darcy observes that:

> You either choose this method of passing the evening because you are in each other's confidence ... or because you are conscious that your figures appear to the greatest

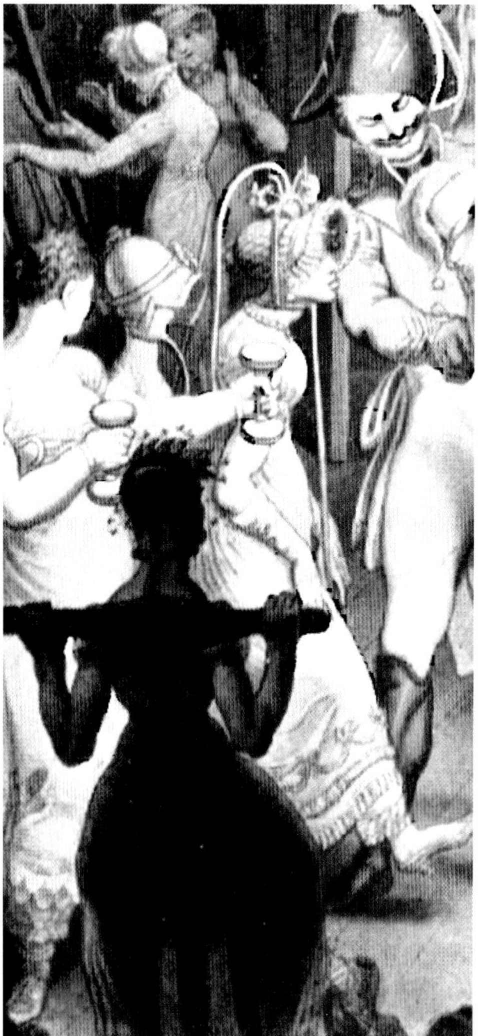

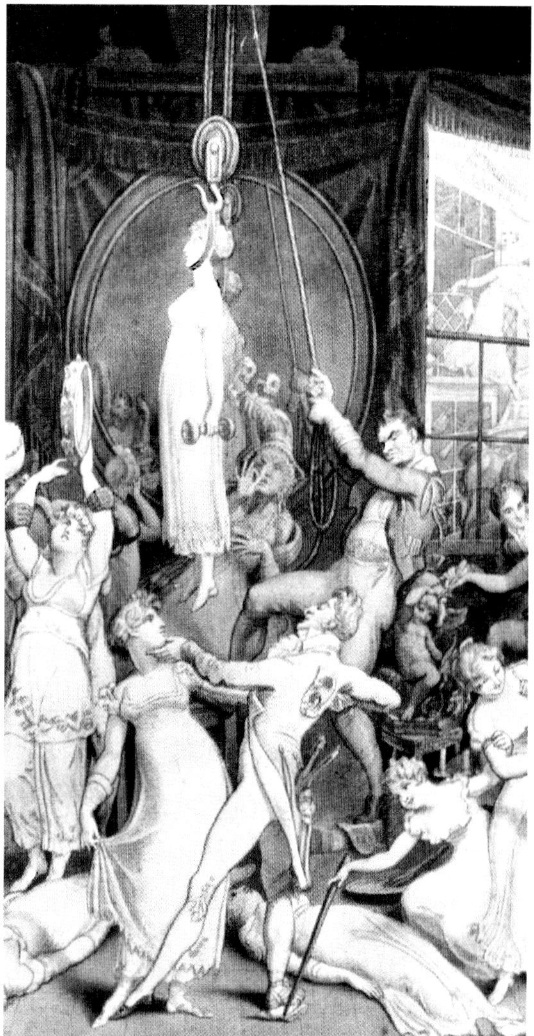

Above left: A young lady sits strapped onto a back board with a collar. In the background, her friends are wearing the London Collar and the Hinkley Collar.

Above right: A young lady subjected to the 'Neck Swing' described: 'I was suspended in a neck-swing, which is merely a tackle and pulley fixed to the ceiling of the room; the pulley is hooked to the head-piece of the collar, and the whole person raised so that the toes only touch the ground'.

> advantage in walking: if the first, I should be completely in your way; and if the second, I can admire you much better as I sit by the fire.

Children were taught to dance from an early age, and even though the minuet was no longer fashionable, it was usually taught as it instilled such grace.

There were many parents who weren't satisfied that grace alone was enough, and as Jane alludes to in *Emma*, there were fashionable Ladies Seminaries 'where young ladies for enormous pay might be screwed out of health and into vanity'.

Under the boarding school regime a great deal of emphasis was put on posture and deportment and it wasn't just walking with a pile of books on your head! Lessons were taken in tall straight-backed Cooper's chairs that were deliberately uncomfortable and overly high so their feet couldn't touch the floor, to ensure that the girls would never slouch or deviate from the correct upright posture. There was also a selection of alarming devices to cure the defects of the figure that doctors claimed were the fault of the mother

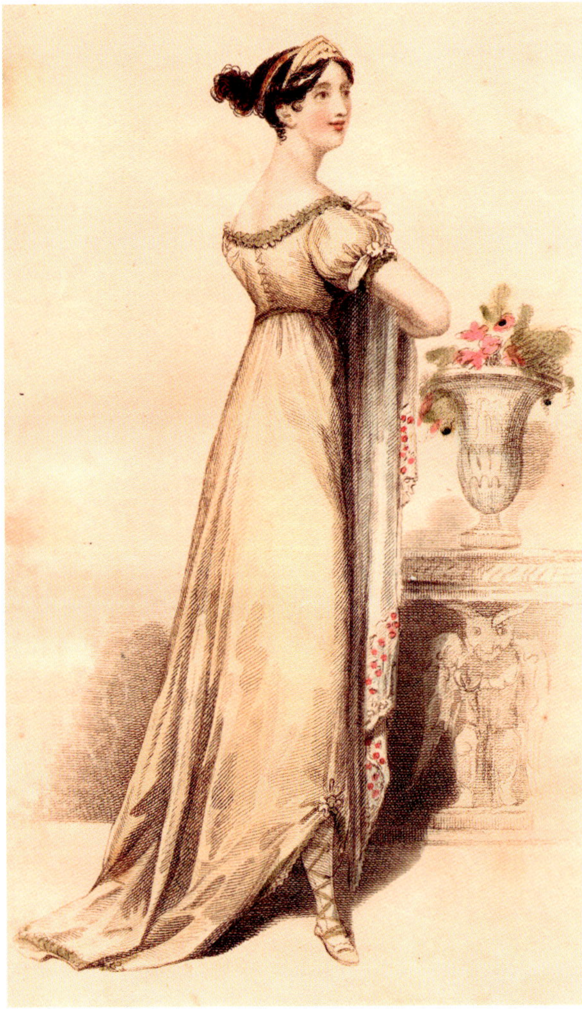

'Evening Dress', *La Belle Assemblée*, February 1813. The young ladies were also placed in mahogany stocks to create the desirable, well-turned ankle with a slightly outturned foot just perfect for these beautiful white satin sandals that lace up above the ankle.

(of course) having swaddled or dressed the child incorrectly during their formative years. Sadly, bent backs and twisted limbs were common, but rather due to illnesses like rickets that were caused by poor nutrition, or childhood injuries never properly healed. There was also a great fear of consumptive diseases, and it was thought that a good upright posture would open the chest and encourage healthy breathing.

There were back boards that were placed in the small of the back with the elbows tied behind these, along with a wooden yoke with leather straps to hold the shoulders, were meant to help straighten and improve the back. A long and elegant neck was particularly important, especially in the first years of the nineteenth century, to complement the fashionable upswept goddess-inspired hairstyles. To achieve this, young ladies were required to wear the 'London Collar' which was a steel rod topped with a 'U'-shaped piece of steel with a sharp edge that came up near to the jaw line ready to wound her if she slouched. Another version was topped with an artificial flower stuck full of pins so that if she bent her head or tucked in her chin rather than maintaining a graceful neck, she would get a face full of pins.

More serious cases might be subject to a variety of metal collars that would force the neck into the correct posture. The Hinkley Collar was an attachment that could be added to a metal back plate high between the shoulder blades supported by steel stays, from which an iron rod rose and curved above the head with leather straps attached to fit around the neck and under the chin to keep the head pulled firmly upwards. Whilst for the truly problematic cases a young lady might be condemned to take lessons lying on her back on the floor, or subjected to Monsieur Le Vacher's Neck Swing, a series of straps to correct the neck and jawline by which she was suspended from the ceiling.

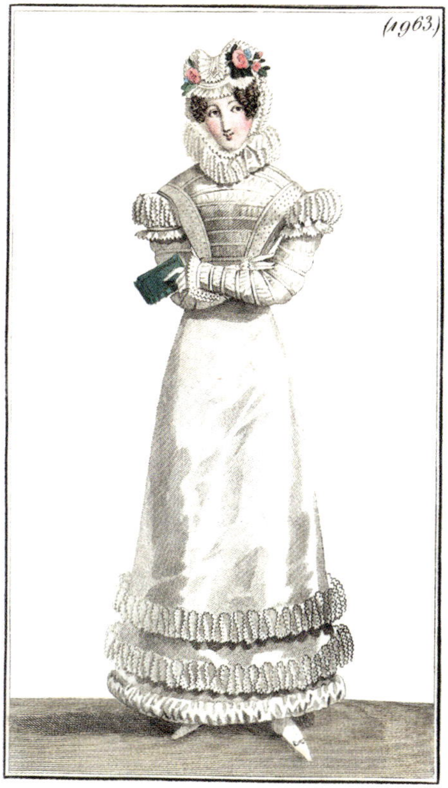

Left: Her white tulle gown is accessorised by a Gothic novel and an array of romantic ruffs. ('Costumes Parisiens', 1821)

Below: 'Tales of Wonder' (James Gillray, 1802), satirising the vogue for 'foolish' female novel reading.

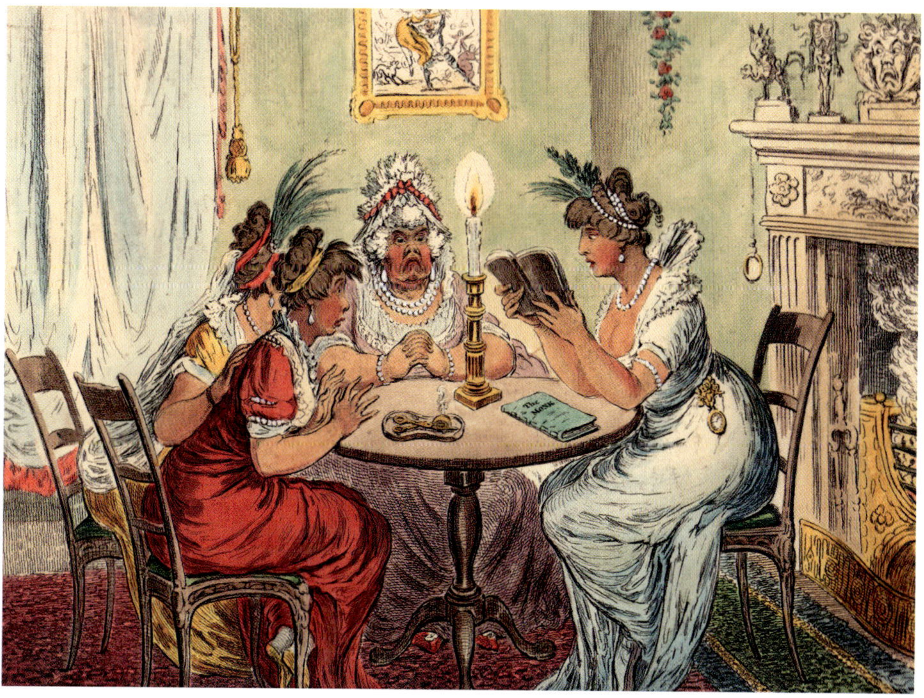

8

Gothic Beauty in the Age of Romance

No family was left untouched by the huge death toll of the Napoleonic Wars, as proportionately more young men were lost in battle during those long years than in the First World War. Having dedicated their entire lives to the prospect of matrimony, in losing their fiancés and beaux women also lost hope for their futures. So many women were in mourning and a complete state of dislocation, not knowing what to do now their prospects were entirely changed and curtailed, so they took solace in literature.

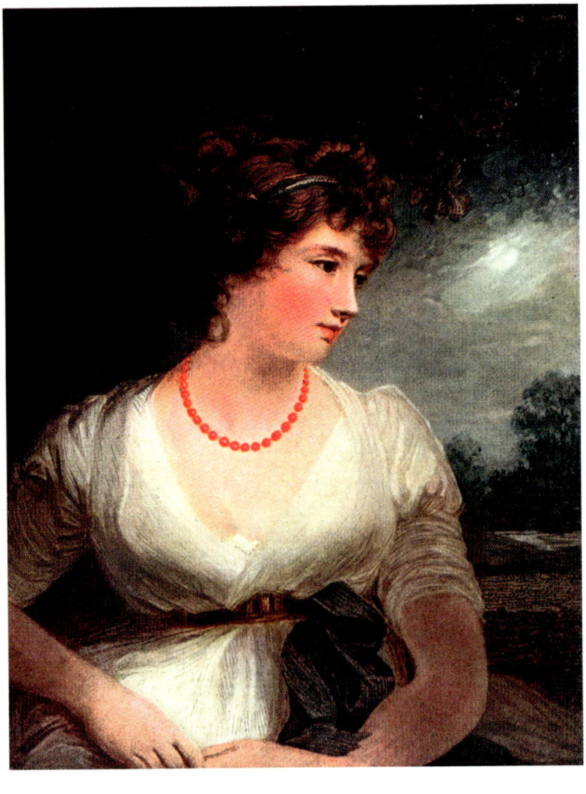

Jane Elizabeth, Countess of Oxford (after John Hoppner, 1797) well met by moonlight.

Gothic novels spoke with a clear female sensitivity, and romantic poetry allowed the heart to leap and plunge. The heroines of Gothic novels were always far too embroiled in mystery to spend too long worried about becoming that most reviled creature – an old maid. They had agency, they had prospects – even if they were dire – and most of all they had enough gumption to be able to solve the mystery that ensnared them and escape the danger that threatened them so that all could safely be restored.

As Jane Austen parodies in *Northanger Abbey*, the idea of women devouring literature to nurture their own thoughts and feelings was deeply controversial and greatly frowned upon. A. F. Crell, the doctor who wrote *The Family Oracle of Health, Economy, Medicine, And Good Living Adapted to All Ranks of Society, From The Palace To The Cottage* in 1824, asserted that: 'We have not a doubt, that the increased demand for the perusal of novels and tales is accountable for much of the prevalence of nervous disorders ... [especially when] poring over them by the midnight lamp, and the consequent robbing of the brain of its healthful measure of sleep'.

There were other dangers too. Goethe's tragic tale of unrequited love *The Sorrows of Young Werther*, published in 1774, had provoked such sensibilities and so many suicides that it was banned in Leipzig in 1775. As was the Werther costume of indigo jacket and yellow waistcoat that became a pan-European vogue as the novel was embraced everywhere. Marianne has shades of Werther in *Sense and Sensibility* and Jane refers directly to the phenomena in *Love and Friendship* when she has Laura encourage Janetta to reject a suitor chosen by her parents because 'he had never read The Sorrows of Werther, and we were certain that Janetta could feel no affection for him, or at least that she ought to feel none'.

Young Werther and his sorrows inspired a slew of poetry, thousands of art prints featuring poor Charlotte grieving for him by a fashionable casket memorial and even a Werther perfume.

Gothic heroines also inspired fashion. Eleanor Tilney in *Northanger Abbey* always wears white because she wants to emulate Emily in *The Mysteries of Udolpho* by one of Jane's contemporary authors, Ann Radcliffe. She and Catherine are obsessed by the tale that sees Emily spend an inordinate amount of time in a white veil being chased through a romantic moonlit ruinous landscape whilst attempting to deflect the evil plans and ungentlemanly intentions of a series of unpleasant relatives and unworthy suitors.

The fashion press concurred, as the *Ladies' Monthly Museum* put it in June 1802: 'the close, all white, shroud looking, ghostly chemise undress of the ladies, who seem to glide like spectres, with their shrouds wrapt tight about their forms'.

La Belle Assemblée confirmed it in 1806, writing: 'wrap them in elegant robes of light impalpable ether'. It was clear that where fashionable white was the sheer and semi-nude drapery of a Grecian statue, Gothic white was an ethereal shroud of multi-layered muslin and moonlight. This was an echo of the tradition of young women being buried in their wedding gowns with a chaplet of white flowers added if they had died before their wedding day.

The gothic glamour of white muslin took on a new incarnation with the rise of the 'Muslin Disease', as doctors called it, blaming the scant gowns worn with little more than an elegant Kashmir shawl even in the dead of winter for the rise of tuberculosis and consumption. It drained vitality from the soul and roses from the cheeks leaving its victims frail and wan. Although a horrible deadly disease, the idea of being delicate, frail and ethereal almost beyond

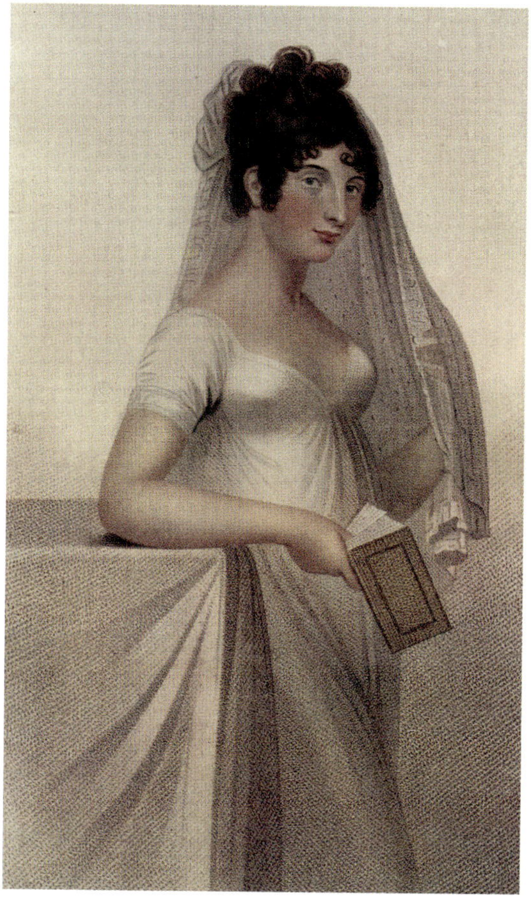

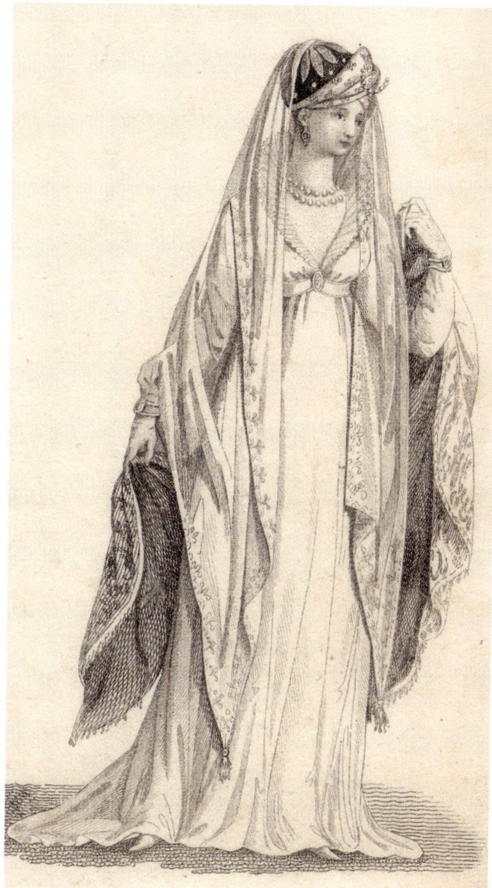

Above left: A portrait of a woman by Adam Buck.

Above right: Parisian fashions, *La Belle Assemblée,* August 1806, depicting the vogue for the long, ethereal veil.

this world seemed terribly romantic, especially given the folkloric belief that the consumptive was forced to spend all night at fairy revels leaving them weak by day, barely able to rise from an elegantly proportioned daybed whilst gradually fading away to the other side.

If a lady wasn't fortunate enough to suffer from such a glamorous illness, she could feign going 'into decline'. The haunted fragile look of a consumptive could, they thought, be simulated by drinking large quantities of vinegar to suppress the appetite and encourage dark circles around the eyes. More scholarly girls would encourage dark, haunted eyes by staying up all night swooning over romantic poetry – especially that written by the devilishly handsome Lord Byron.

Consumption destroyed the appetite as it provoked radical weight loss, leaving the sufferer slender and pale, able only to face tiny meals such as a saucer of strawberries or cherries. Such romantic fruits would also encourage pretty, reddened lips even if they did belie the gastrointestinal distress the illness was causing.

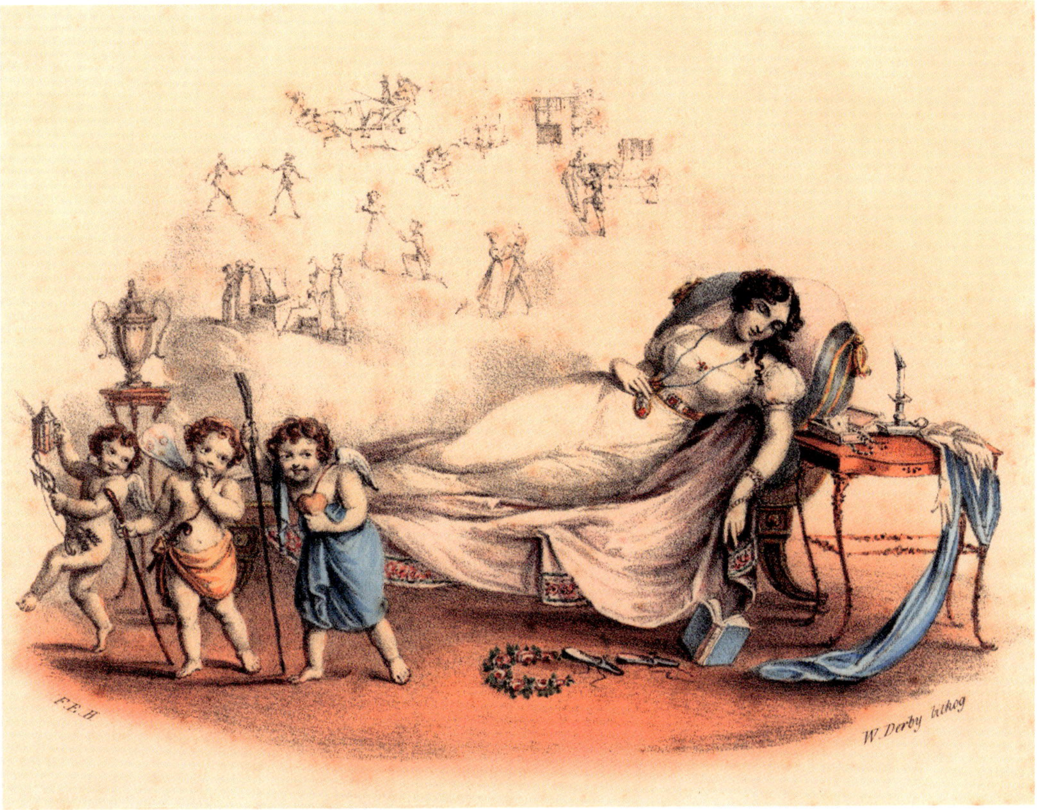

'Heart Stealing' (W. Derby, *c.* 1820). A young woman dreams of romance and adventure inspired by 'unhealthy' Gothic literature.

Lord Byron wrote the immortal lines of 'She Walks in Beauty' on 12 June 1814 after meeting his cousin's young wife, the botanist Anne Beatrix Wilmot-Horton, at a party the night before:

> She walks in beauty, like the night
> Of cloudless climes and starry skies;
> And all that's best of dark and bright
> Meet in her aspect and her eyes;
> Thus mellowed to that tender light
> Which heaven to gaudy day denies.

She was wearing a black spangled mourning gown that contrasted beautifully with her pale complexion and 'every raven tress' of her hair. Just how her eyes were 'dark and bright' is not recorded but there were those who resorted to belladonna ('beautiful lady'), a derivative of deadly nightshade, to create the beautiful limpid eyes that spoke so eloquently of a soul full of passion. The ladies of the Renaissance used a feather to drop a small amount into each eye to create the desired effect. Unfortunately, with recent advances in ocular surgery

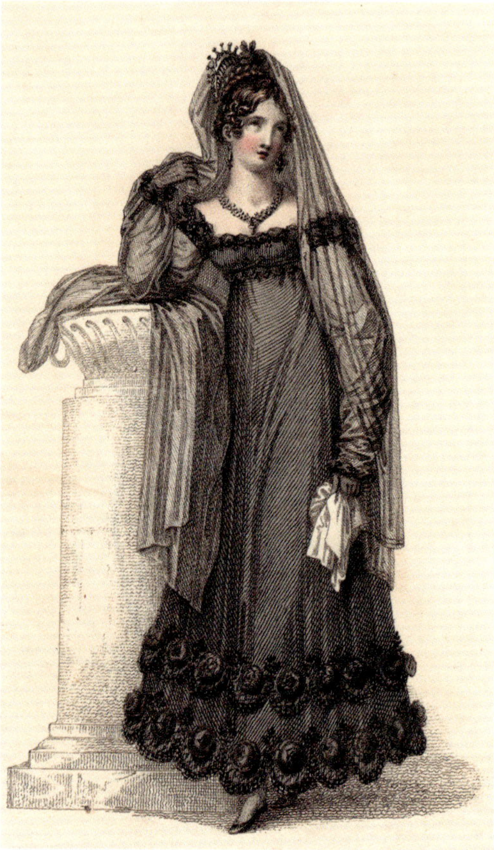

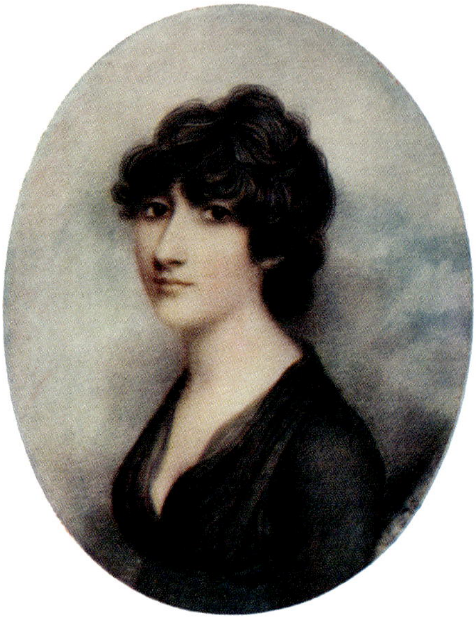

Above: The mesmerising dark, haunted eyes of Elizabeth Ellis (portrait miniature by Andrew Plimer, *c.* 1810).

Left: 'Full Mourning Evening Dress', Ackermann's *Repository of Arts*, December 1818.

facilitated by the use of belladonna to open the pupil, to the Regency mind, belladonna was freshly renewed with scientific credentials to countermand any hint that the deadly poison might compromise eye health, potentially causing blindness and paralysis.

In 1825 *The Family Oracle of Health* suggested the use of belladonna: 'A very little of it rubbed on the eye-lids will in a short time enlarge the pupil to a wonderful degree, and the effect will continue for some hours.' They did, however, caution not to use too much 'least it make the pupils too large and staring'.

Far safer was 'the Circassian method' of beautifying the eye which the author of *The Family Oracle* advocated strongly as both non-injurious and free from expense, citing Lord Byron as having 'hung some of his finest gems on a beautiful eye-lash'.

The Circassian method was popular in Circassia, Georgia, and Persia where the women were renowned for their beauty because their diligent mothers were at great pains to nurture their beautiful eyelashes by routinely snipping off the tips every six weeks from the time they were babies. This would promote them growing long and glossy.

Once you had mastered the Circassian method, if your lashes still needed further enhancement you could try another beautifier from the Middle East and darken your lashes with antimony: 'which is put both on the hairs and at the skin at their roots, while a small streak of it is often extended outwards from the exterior angle of each eye'.

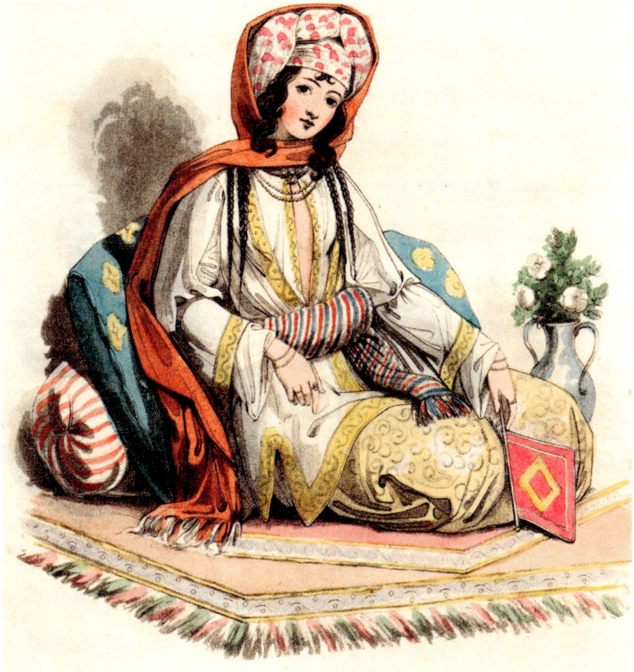

'The Fair Circassian', *The Lady's Magazine*, May 1819. Her visit to London with the Persian Ambassador in 1819 was widely reported as everyone was entranced by her marvellous complexion and beautiful eyes.

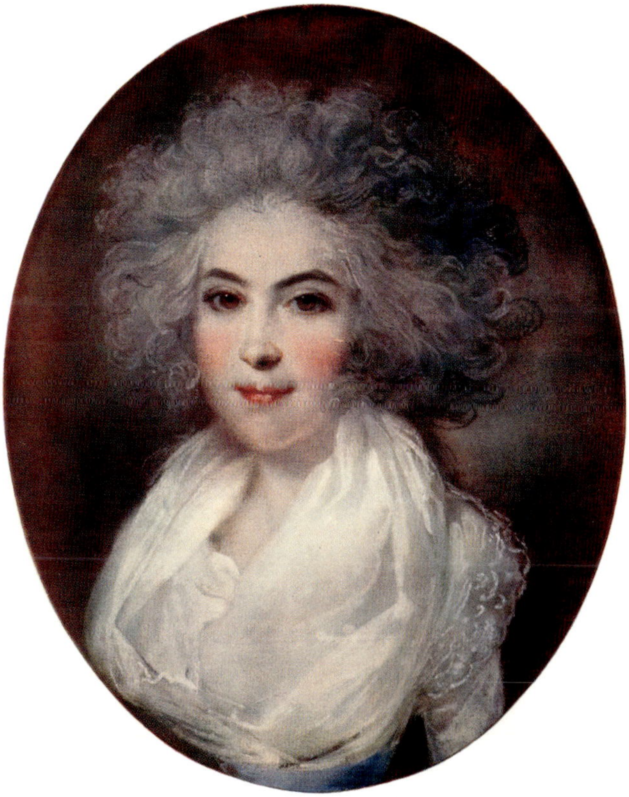

Portrait of Mrs Thomas Raikes (John Russell RA). She has beautifully mastered the art of make-up, especially enchanting eyeliner.

If you could not get antimony kohl, you could try their recipe for charred frankincense mixed with the juice of elderberries or the simple bedroom expedient of lampblack. This was gathered by holding a clean saucer over the flame of your bedside candle to gather the soot. This could be mixed with a drop of almond oil, a tiny amount of pomade or wax and smoothed onto the upper lashes in gentle upward strokes using a paintbrush from your watercolour set. You might also use an ivory bodkin from your sewing box as this bore a striking resemblance to the traditional ivory or olive wood wand used in the East.

Without any contemporary references for confirmation, it seems unlikely that such a strong look appeared in many drawing rooms here. It is far more likely that the British Fair applied it more delicately with a narrow line painted tightly to and between the lashes to do no more than enhance and shade. An alternative was burnt frankincense which gave a colour that was more brown than black and possibly more suitable for those with pale eyes, especially if maintaining the fiction of natural beauty.

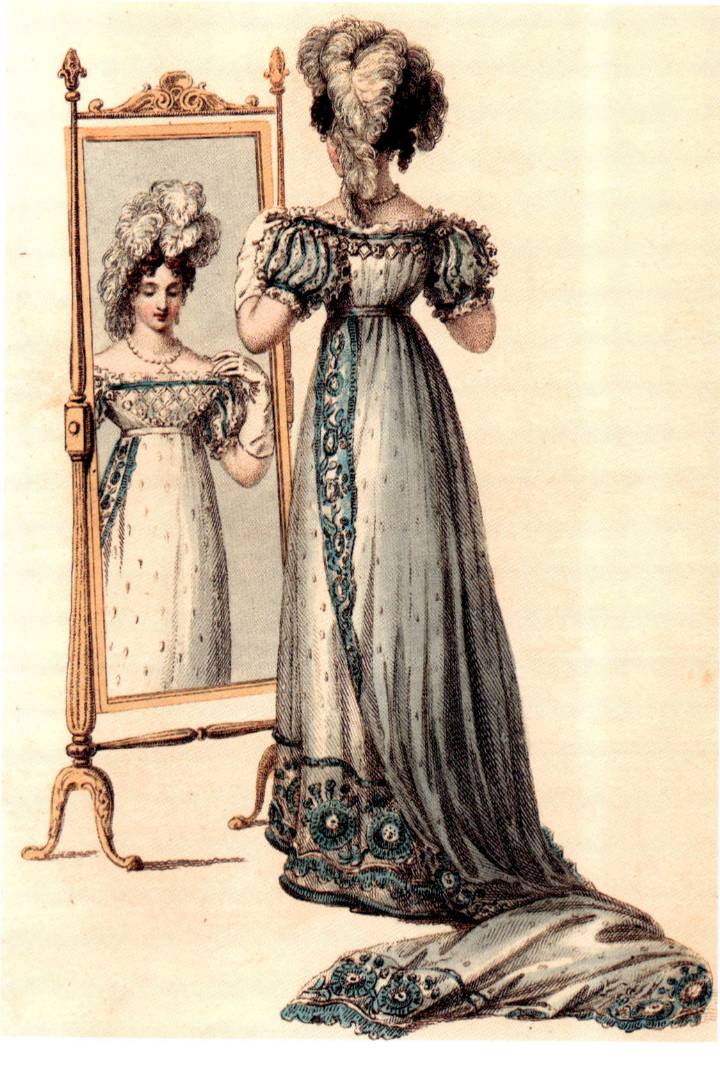

'Court Dress', Ackermann's *Repository of Arts*, September 1822.